Alt-Vet

The Revolutionary Pet Care and Longevity Solution

DR. MITSIE VARGAS

Certified Traditional Chinese Veterinary Medicine Practitioner

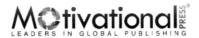

MOtivational PRESS

LEADERS IN GLOBAL PUBLISHING

Published by Motivational Press, Inc.
1777 Aurora Road
Melbourne, Florida, 32935
www.MotivationalPress.com

Manufactured in the United States of America.

ISBN: 978-1-62865-392-2

CONTENTS

• • • •

FOREWORD

· · · ·

I AM SO HONORED AND HAPPY to have read Dr. Mitsie Vargas' new manuscript entitled "Alt-Vet". I totally agree with what Dr. Vargas states in this book "**it is your pet and your choice**". Making a good choice can be a challenge. after reading this exciting and informative book though, you gain a better understanding of the holistic approach to medical care, prevention and treatment of a pet, and, in turn, making a sound choice for your own pet.

From the Traditional Chinese Veterinary Medicine, a clinician needs to have a good disposition, passion, and the intention to heal in order to bring the "good Qi" and become a successful practitioner. It was obvious to me that Dr. Vargas has those qualities along with a desire to teach others. She is one of the best teacher assistants at the Chi Institute that has trained nearly 6,000 veterinarians to provide TCVM care for pets in over 50 countries around the world since established in 1998. It is from that desire to teach TCVM concepts that this book was born. Whereas my path is to teach TCVM to veterinarians, Dr. Vargas' is to teach TCVM basic concepts to pet caregivers.

The concepts discussed here will appear revolutionary, yet they are based on time-honored healing methods and principles that have been re-interpreted using modern technology and science. The idea of balance in everything is the root of TCVM and these concepts should be taken in that same vein. This book's intention is to open the eyes of many owners whether their pets are facing a grim prognosis or they are new to pet ownership and are in need of direction. They should seek a veterinarian knowledgeable in TCVM to help them institute the advice given here.

I know Dr. Vargas has poured the same passion and dedication shown in her studies at Chi institute and has imbued this book with good healing Qi.

May this book bring the answers you seek and may the good Qi be with you always,

Huisheng Xie, DVM MS PhD

Clinical Associate Professor, Integrative Medicine Service, College of Veterinary Medicine, University of Florida, Gainesville, Florida

Professor and Dean of the Chi Institute, Reddick, Florida

www.tcvm.com

PREFACE

• • • •

THIS BOOK HAS BEEN A LABOR of love that has kept me on my toes for over a year. I am so thankful to my husband Gaston for being so patient with me, especially when I was immersed in my writing spells and forgetting that life kept going on around me. He truly is my rock and the love of my life. I am also very thankful to my two wonderful daughters Victoria and Angelica for their understanding and cooperation. They've become my biggest fans and I adore them. I cannot forget to thank my beta readers, my sister Melissa and my niece Andrea, for their support and feedback (they are the toughest grammar police out there). I have to say that my dad Teo also deserves my acknowledgement for being my guinea pig taking my herbal advice and believing in me.

I would like to honor my grandmother Juana Davila's memory by saying she was a great influence in my life and a great example of being in tune with natural healing. I would also like to honor my mother Margie's memory for teaching me about work ethic and encouraging my dream to become a veterinarian.

I need to thank my friend and mentor Dr. Huisheng Xie for his kind encouragement and praise. It is thanks to his willingness to share his expertise and his passion that I have enjoyed my journey to becoming a certified TCVM practitioner.

It would be a crime not to mention my friend and editor extraordinaire John Peragine, whose grammar skills and helpful attitude made my ideas and revolutionary concepts become understandable and accessible to all.

I have to also mention my friend and animal behaviorist Marco Magiolo, for his support and advice for this book. I owe thanks to my dear friend Lisa Baker for being my earliest supporter of this project and for working tirelessly for the wellbeing of animals in our county.

I also have to thank my patients and their owners because they are my greatest teachers. The trust they put in my hands is a humbling honor and I will strive to always give them 100% of my capabilities and love. This book is a way to help even those pet owners across the world, which I haven't had the pleasure of meeting, they deserve to know that there are alternative options to care for their pets.

Finally, I must say that I'm thankful to all the pets I've had the pleasure to share my life with because they have shaped who I am as a veterinarian.

In my quest to keep them with me as long as possible, I started my journey into a holistic approach to medicine. The reality is that I am an acupuncturist today because I was attempting to keep my beloved German Shepherds out of pain. I've always had second-hand dogs or strays for pets. They became more than mere companions; they were my avatars and friends. I'd like to share my adoption story of a senior dog we named Sam, a seven-year old German Shepherd who changed my life. In 1997, I had a one-year old German Shepherd named Bruno who was a very hyper and energetic guy and I felt he needed a friend other than our 4 cats. I told my dear friend Lisa, the Executive Director of the Humane Society of Polk, to put my name on a waiting list for the next "German Shepherd-ish" dog under a year old that would come in the shelter.

Lisa called a couple of weeks later to tell me that a five-month old beautiful puppy had been relinquished because the owners did not have enough time for him. I was busy with my incipient little practice, so I sent my husband to pick up our new puppy. Imagine my surprise, when he came home with a mangy, forty-nine pound, tick and flea infested wolf hybrid looking older dog. I asked him what happened and he said this guy was on death row and was staring at him begging to be saved. The dog turned his face toward me and in that moment I felt a deep connection to his brandy colored eyes. That was it for me and I welcomed him into my heart.

It took us three months to get him healthy enough to meet our Bruno. In their first meeting, they had an awful fight. This terrified me because I was already so invested in Sam that I could not take it if he wouldn't fit in our pack. To my relief, from then on they became best friends. We were blessed to have Sam for an amazing nine years! I learned so much about supplements, nutrition and alternative medicine trying to manage his arthritis and old age issues but, alas, he was not immortal. He died of an embolism while running into my husband's arms. His last day was spent at the pool bossing around our two other German Shepherds Bruno and Hans.

Cats have been lifelong sidekicks, confidants, and bed warmers for me. There are several special ones that had shaped my views on vaccination, behavior issues, declawing, and the importance of food. Most of them lived an average of 15 years and were pretty healthy. Currently, I am a proud foster failure of three adorable kitties; Keanu, Texas and Charlie. They keep me entertained with their antics and are teaching me all about cat development. I blame any typos in this book on these rambunctious kitties because they tried to edit the book every time they saw me at the computer. I am also the staff, feeder, and occasional petter of my feral friend Tom.

Another great animal teacher was my beloved dog Hans. He came to me as a second hand dog too. He was nine months when the owner left him at my clinic. His owner was a nurse working twelve hour shifts and leaving Hans in a cage all that time. Hans, sweet as he was, , was totally unsocialized, did not know any commands, was not potty trained or neutered, severely underweight, and extremely anxious and needy.

Within two weeks of having him, we successfully potty trained him and taught him to sit and stay. Teaching him to walk on a leash and to interact with our other dogs and the cats was another story. I had to leave him out at doggy camp for ten days for rigorous obedience training. We also worked with his trainer for six weeks in order to fix his more destructive and aggressive tendencies.

It took time, but he ended up being a very loved member of our family for ten years. I learned so much about dog training and behavior from him! We were never able to take Hans' prey instinct out of him, but he accepted our pug Daisy as his companion when my other German Shepherd Bruno passed away. That was a big triumph because, prior to that, anything smaller than him was game! His anxiety levels disappeared until he hit his senior years. At that time, I put a Gold implant on his acupuncture point for anxiety and he improved 90%. I am proud to say he lived a happy, healthy life after his traumatic first nine months. Even years after Hans' death, I still miss him terribly! He was the one dog that grew up with my girls, always protective of his pack and always a good listener.Nowadays, I happen to have two Pugs and a White German Shepherd. The Pugs came from less than stellar circumstances. Daisy was the runt of the litter and I traded the treatment of her sick littermates for her ownership. I knew she needed nose surgery and some special care. I had a giant hole in my heart from losing my dog Bruno, so she really helped me through the grieving process. She has been a sweet, friendly, and loving companion. She even posed for the Tui-na pictures in the massage chapter.

'Puppy' is the dog on the cover of this book. He was dumped at the Humane Society and Lisa (executive director and friend) knew I would fall in love with his quirky, hyper personality. He is a perennial puppy and a destructive force, but such a loving dog that we can't help but to put up with his crazy energy. He has been a handful, but I wouldn't trade any of the things he has destroyed for him. He is my personal comedian and keeps me laughing every day. When I broke my leg, he showed a side I never knew existed. He was my devoted lap companion and the sweetest nurse. He would lay over my broken leg and tried licking it all the time. He even enjoyed riding in the wheelchair! He is living proof that all pets have the potential to be wonderful companions.

Ulrich, the white Shepherd, is the baby of the family and going to be a service dog for my daughter. As such, he will undergo extensive specialized training, but for now he worked as my model for the emergency points illustration.

If even one pet is saved by the advice in this book, then my intention is fulfilled. I hope you learn something new, that you open your mind to alternative medicine, and that you find something here that will help your pet live a longer, healthier and happier life.

Mitsie Vargas, DVM, CVA

Winter Haven, FL

September 2016

CHAPTER 1

THE HOLISTIC VIEW

• • • •

Have you ever considered taking away a leg or another part of your pet that was unhealthy? If your dog or cat was a car, you wouldn't hesitate to replace the malfunctioning parts for new ones, would you?

We know our beloved pets are not machines, so why treat them like cars when it comes to their health? My profession as a licensed veterinarian follows the human evidence-based model of practice. In veterinary school, we are taught the allopathic medicine system of using drugs or remedies to cure any ill. It is a mechanistic approach that views animal bodies as machines and disease as a broken mechanism in the system. In that model, you take the broken parts away with surgery or add temporary solutions such as drug therapy.

I am part of a growing group of veterinarians that are upgrading the rigid, mechanistic-only approach and embracing alternative ways of looking at animal bodies in a holistic (whole-body) method. We see animals as living ecosystems. All their organs are connected by an invisible energy that is the life force of your pet.

Suppose you see an animal that has passed. What is the difference between being alive and not alive? The pet is there, but there is a vital energy that gives it life and a personality. Without that force coursing through the animal, it will begin to break down into the elemental building blocks of all material things, living or nonliving.

Holistic medicine is based on the concept that we are all made of energy and that energy has organization. This realization is not "hot from the press news" though; the Chinese developed the concept of *Yin & Yang* (two opposing, but complementing forces of energy) over five thousand years ago! Other ancient civilizations developed similar whole body health systems based on the idea that all living things are essentially made of energy.

Why is present-day Western society hesitant to embrace these holistic modalities? If alternative medicine was a passing fad, it would have disappeared long ago. There is a lot of misinformation online about pet care issues. The majority of pet owners are completely unaware they can help their pets live longer and enjoy healthier lives. Hence, I have decided to share my experiences and knowledge in this book. It is truly the story of how alternative medicine works miracles of healing on a daily basis.When a pet is in pain or has a cancerous tumor, I suspect a disruption of the energy flow and a disharmony among the body systems. As a holistic practitioner, I also believe in a strong interaction of the mind with the body. When there is balance between the two, healing can occur.

In your pet's body, there is a community in which one organ's health can affect the function of other body systems. Like a falling domino chain reaction, one failing organ can bring about the eventual failure of the entire body.

One of the components not emphasized in allopathic, modern-day, Western veterinary medicine, is how the mental and emotional state of your pet effects not only the health and wellbeing of your pet, but also in the healing process. In standard veterinary medicine, there is belief that animals don't have emotions like humans do. From many years of experience, I'm here to tell you that animals have feelings too! They carry emotional baggage and have mental illnesses similar to our own. I can't begin to calculate the vast number of bipolar cats and schizophrenic dogs I've treated in my career.

The environmental and mental state of the pet can speed or delay recovery. In many cases, the mental or emotional state of the owners can transfer to their pet and becomes a factor in their pet's healing.

Animal trainers know how much the emotional state of a pet owner has a direct bearing on the response of the pet. They emphasize the state of mind of the owner first, before even teaching the initial commands. They know that being calm and assertive when training animals is important because they somehow receive your feelings and act accordingly. It is not a giant leap to surmise that a worried pet owner, convinced the worst is going to happen, maydelay their pet's healing by making them nervous or stressed.

Skeptics might ask what role could mind or mental therapy have with animals. I will categorically answer that the mental and emotional balance of pets affects their health in many ways. Considering the many pet abuse cases I have seen, in my experience I have seen a disproportionate number of them acquire liver or heart disease. In TCVM, the explanation for this phenomena is that traumatic events and grief cause *Qi* blockages in the Liver, where *Qi* is stored. There is also the heart to consider. In TCVM, the heart is the emperor and storage for the spirit and mind (*Shen*). When there is a *Shen* disturbance, it manifests in abnormal behavior or disease of the physical heart. Having a loving, stable home full of positive mental stimulation can aid our animals companions recovery and in disease prevention.

In regards to the environment, there are many levels in which it affects the health of our pets. First, the degree of pollution greatly diminishes their quality of life. For example, cigarette smoke exposure (whether second or third hand) can cause an array of physical problems including, but not limited to, cancer, asthma, lung issues and allergic skin disease.

Secondly, the seasons follow the Five Element Theory. This theory categorizes five primordial elements (Wood, Fire, Earth, Metal and Water) with a different set of characteristics and energies that permeate through the whole Universe. It is also in constant interaction with the energetic field of your pet's body. Seasonality is then a big factor in disease processes, depending on which element dominates that time of the year and the Meridians it affects.

HOW DO ALLOPATHIC AND ALTERNATIVE VETERINARY MEDICINE DIFFER?

The main distinction between the two is how they approach the concept of health and wellness. Allopathic tends toward a cookie cutter approach; there is one cure for each illness across the pet population. The main flaw of that approach is that dogs are not cookies. Consider the tale of two different Golden Retrievers that came to me because the owners said they were urinating in the house. Neither dog had a urinary infection as determined by the standard laboratory tests. One was a one year old (Lucy) and the other a twelve year old spayed female (Stella). According to the traditional Western approach, both would've undergone a battery of tests and put on a potent medication called PROIN. What many pet owners don't know is that the active ingredient in PROIN fell out of human use due to severe side effects including kidney failure. I am an integrative practitioner. After running my standard tests to rule out infections, masses, and bladder stones, I diagnose using Traditional Chinese Veterinary Medicine (TCVM) principles.

A TCVM practitioner assesses the personality of the pet based on the Five Element Theory. Once that is determined, then a pattern of diseases can be assumed based on the relationship of the pet personality with the Meridian (energy system) affected.

Imagine the body as having a number of roadways, a kind of super-highway of energy. The roads connect to different organ systems in the body. The configuration of the roadways is affected by the personality (One of Five Elements) of the pet.

Think of it this way: Metropolitan cities have many similarities. They have shops, businesses, places of entertainment, utilities, and so forth. Think of each of those as an organ system. The road configuration within cities is essentially the same; they form a grid. However, the grid in Miami is different than New York's which is different than Boston's. Each city has its own personality, complete with strengths and weaknesses. One strength of New York is the fantastic, moving water that comes from aqueducts upstate. In New Orleans, a weakness (possible disease) is that it is prone to flooding and stagnation.

When I do my assessment on a pet, I determine what their body systems strengths and vulnerabilities are based upon their personality.

Roads within a city allow people, services, and items that are necessary for the population to survive. A fish market needs fish. A hospital needs medical equipment and supplies. When the roads are open and functioning correctly, everything runs smoothly, and merchandise and people arrive where they need to go. There is a constant flow of energy and a daily routine in most cities.

What happens if there is a traffic jam? A damaged bridge? A traffic accident? The flow is interrupted. When the flow is damaged or blocked, the businesses, and people are negatively affected. The longer the blockage, the more profound the effect. Eventually, a business will close if the problem is not remedied and whole communities can shut down.

This is a simplistic model for the energy in the body. The roads are called Meridians, while the flow of nutrient, and energy is *Qi*. TCVM practice allows me to identify where the blockages are and release them.

Consider it from a completely medical-allopathic point of view. If blood stops flowing in your body, you will die. If your spinal cord is severed, then anything below that break will no longer function because energy can no longer flow through nerve cells. If oxygen stops flowing to the brain, it will begin to die. The longer the flow is cut, the more sections of the brain will perish until there is total system failure.

At the deepest and most basic level, your pet's body is made of energy or *Qi*. According to TCVM principles, your pet is born with a certain amount of source energy or *Jing Qi*. This is transmitted by the genes and stored in the kidneys. That energy gets depleted with disease and normal wear and tear of the body. The only other sources of energy come from the Universal / Environment (*Qing Qi*) and the energy from food (*Gu Qi*). Therefore, food can be used to restore the deficient energy levels caused by disease. This view of the importance of food in healing is a universal concept made famous by the father of Modern Medicine (Hippocrates) when he uttered the saying, "Let food be thy medicine".

Interestingly, when I see a patient with congenital diseases, I put most of the emphasis of my treatment in the food or *Gu Qi*. I do this because Iknow that this patient was born with a low level of *Jing Qi*. Food therapy, using the energetic properties of each food item and their benefits, is crucial for premature puppies and kitties or those who did not receive enough colostrum. It is my experience that *Jing Qi* has a strong correlation with longevity. The best example is when I see inbred or "puppy mill" dogs that have multiple congenital issues and a weak immune system in general. If these poor souls do not receive proper care, they will simply perish at an early age. Conversely, with good care, a nurturing home environment, and great quality diet supplemented with herbals and other appropriate nutraceuticals, these animals can live a longer and better quality life.

Confused yet? Don't worry! I am planning on an in depth discussion of each modality of TCVM in later chapters. For now, however, it's safe to say that the practitioner will NOT be looking at urinary incontinence as a one issue disease. They will be looking at it as a symptom of a root problem arising from an imbalance of energy along a major Meridian.

Although standard drugs might be used, the patient would also be treated using acupuncture and herbal and food recommendations. The goal of integrated medicine is to improve not only the issue at hand, but the overall health of the patient.

The Golden Retrievers in the previous story were quite different. Lucy was a Fire personality and Stella an Earth personality. When I felt their pulses, they were diametrically opposed; one was strong, fast, and superficial while the other one weak and deep. Their tongues were quite different too. Lucy's was red and Stella's was pale with some lavender in it. This information provided the guidance I needed to diagnose.

Lucy had an excess condition caused by a diet too hot energetically for her personality constitution. Moving down from the north to hot Florida and eating a dry chicken based kibble were not helping her. Stella had a deficiency in *Qi* due to her age. Both were successfully treated with acupuncture and herbs, but with completely different formulas and points.

Holistic medicine looks for the underlying disharmony causing the symptom. Using a wide array of treatment modalities, this supports the patient to heal thyself. The emphasis is placed in providing the immune system the tools it needs to fix the problem. Consider again our city analogy. The city officials send out work crews to repair roads, bridges, and other structures, while at the same time protecting them from storms, erosion, rust, and even invasive plant species that can take over an area (like cancer). The allopathic approach would be to use dynamite to blow up a road and start over or just set all the plants on fire (chemo and radiation). The problem with this approach is it can hurt other structures because explosives and fires do not differentiate good structures from bad ones.

I treat a lot of pets who have cancer with herbs and diet. In most cases, they get to live a pleasurable, extended, and better quality life than they would have without treatment or, in some cases, as an add on to chemotherapy. The cherry on top is that treating with herbs and acupuncture is lot more cost effective for the owner than some conventional options.

What happens if you have a pet that is prescribed a medication, but cannot get them to take it because they have mastered spitting them out? Many times veterinarians may give pet owners a way to trick the animal into complying, but offer no additional solutions. If the pet does not swallow the pill, they are just out of luck.

Cats are notorious for their pill-spitting abilities. These finicky patients can benefit from food therapy or acupuncture. It is not strange to see my patients undergo a hundred and eighty-degree health and wellness shift once they begin alternative medicine treatments.

The strength of the Holistic approach is in prevention of disease and management of chronic illness with the overall goal of improving quality of life. Can it heal all pets? No, but it can certainly help a large number of them live pain free, happier, and in many cases, longer lives.

NO ANIMAL DIES WITHOUT TRYING ACUPUNCTURE

The first year I started practicing acupuncture, most of my cases were euthanasia appointments. Euthanasia consults are emotionally charged office visits where the owners bring in pets for me to evaluate if there is enough quality of life present to continue care. Sometimes, if the disease toll is such, the most humane course of action is to say goodbye. The process entails administering an overdose of anesthetic so that the pet gently passes away.

I would look at the pet's eyes as they came in, and, if there was a spark and coherence present, I would then ask the clients how they felt about the decision. As it happened, most (9 out 10) would say that they were not ready, but did not know what else to do to make the pet's lives better. I would offer them a free trial of three acupuncture sessions. If they did not see any improvement, then it was likely nothing would change and confirmed that their time was up.

One of those cases was a ten year old Rottweiler named Brandy. She was unable to get up and would snap at her owners out of pain. They were devastated about their decision, so I offered to try at least one session and keep her overnight to observe if there was any improvement. They had never heard of acupuncture and were skeptical, but gave it a chance just to know they had tried everything. The owners said their goodbyes to Brandy and signed all the paperwork to euthanize her in the morning if the session did not help fix her pain.

I have to admit I went overboard and put a lot of needles; Brandy looked like a porcupine. Assertively, I connected many needles to my electro acupuncture unit to provide extra stimulation. That day I was working by myself and had an emergency walk-in. Knowing that Brandy was paralyzed and wouldn't move, I left her on the floor of my comfort room with all the leads attached to the machine (with it timed to go off at thirty minutes). Imagine my surprise when forty five minutes later, while I was still working on that emergency case, I saw Brandy dragging the electro acupuncture machine down the hall. Not only was Brandy able to walk, but she opened the door and greeted us with a look of joy and determination.

I did not tell the owner about the incident, only that Brandy had shown some improvement. I reasoned that it was impossible to sustain this degree of recovery and that maybe in the morning she would relapse. Instead, to my amazement, she was standing on her back legs trying to get out of the kennel that morning. Inspired, she became my beacon of hope for all "terminal" patients. From that moment on, I said to myself, **"No animal dies without trying acupuncture".**

I hope that I have not painted the picture that I am against Western Medicine, because I am not. I just happen to believe in the strength of Allopathic Medicine for handling acute disease due to lack of long term results from drugs and surgery, which provide rapid short term results. Sadly, the advantage weakens with time as these drugs cause other health issues from their side effects. This is sometimes called "the slash and burn" approach.

If there is a fire that is out of control in a forest, fire fighters will often start small fires (backfires) to stop the larger fire from spreading. Sometimes a cancer is so aggressive that only an Allopathic treatment like chemotherapy will work to stop its progress. The problem is that it may not totally stop the cancer and it is deadly to all tissues it comes in contact with. Alternative therapies help in two ways. First, they can address and heal the root cause of the cancer and can spread the healing of damaged tissues from Allopathic treatments. Allopathic and alternative medical treatments work best when administered in tandem, rather than individual silos.

If my pet was hit by a car, I would want him or her to receive pain medication, diagnostics, and anti-inflammatories as soon as possible. I would also want to surgically repair any damage as thoroughly as possible. If I had access to an anti-bleeding herb called Yunnan Bai Yao, I would gladly give it to my pet immediately and later in the recovery phase. However, after the crisis is over, I would turn to TCVM and other alternative healing modalities to speed the healing process. I wouldn't want to manage chronic pain with harmful drugs and would rely on Acupuncture to improve my pet's overall functions.

Food, environment, and personality/mind all contribute to a harmonious state of health. Holistic medicine incorporates these when trying to restore balance to the whole body in the midst of disease. I will highlight all of these topics because total health cannot be achieved if we do not take into account all factors affecting the performance of your pet's body systems.

WHY ISN'T TCVM THE HOLY GRAIL OF VETERINARY MEDICINE?

The allopathic treatment style has been the standard since 1761, when the first school of veterinary medicine opened in Lyon, France. The first veterinary college in the states opened in 1876, in Cornell, New York.

A few hundred years of trial and error pales in comparison to the healing practices of ancient civilizations, like the Chinese, who created volumes of books dedicated just to acupuncture and herbal remedies in horses. They created those texts over two millennia ago, and are still in use today.

China was not the only nation with early roots in veterinary medicine. In India, ancient healers wrote texts on treating animals using Ayurveda. This system of healing was originally developed for humans and relies on the use of herbs, massage, and meditation to increase longevity. That modality is like a cousin to TCVM because it also uses the Five elements and pet body type to prescribe medicines and diets with the aim of preventing diseases inherent in their body shapes.

While TCVM is becoming more recognized in the US, the use of Ayurvedic veterinary medicine is still inceptive. Curiously, the majority of veterinarians and pet owners assume Alternative Animal Medicine is a new fad, pursued by hipster owners on a whim of special treatment for their animal companions. While the exposure in mainstream media may be on the rise as something new, the actual practices are very old. The key to making TCVM and alternative pet medicine more popular lies in incorporating it into the established Western Medicine model. This collaborative approach has been proven to have better outcomes than treating with only alternative or western approaches exclusively.

The WHO director general Dr. Margaret Chan in her 2014-2023 Directives established that Complementary or Traditional Medicine is not only an effective way to offer healthcare, but a necessary one. Her goals are:

1. Building the knowledge base and formulating national policies for the use of Traditional Chinese Veterinary Medicine.

2. Strengthening safety, quality, and effectiveness through regulation.

3. Promoting universal health coverage by integrating TCVM services and self-health care into national health systems.

I strongly believe this world trend of pursuing Integrative Medicine extends to pet owners and animal lovers who want to explore all options of care for their beloved companions.

I've heard other alternative medicine practitioners verbalize a deep seated belief that "big pharma" will never allow TCVM, or any alternative medicine system, to get too big or threaten the billion dollar industry of veterinary pharmacology. Although the pharmaceutical industry appears to have a very profitable animal related business, I do not ascribe to the notion that they want to suppress alternative medicine practices.

In part, it is hard for me to believe that the veterinary industry would put greed and profits ahead of patient care and wellbeing. Historically, veterinarians have been one of the most trusted professions and that reputation is well earned. We put in many hours of study and make a lot of sacrifices to enter a profession that is not as financially rewarding as related human medicine fields.

Many of us working in the animal health field get remunerated with the deep satisfaction in our ability to make a difference or save the life of an animal.

Of course, we still have bills to pay including continuing education, licenses, support staff, medicine, supplies, equipment, and taxes in order to function as a business. Quality veterinary services take time and have a dedicated staff, which all translates into a higher costs. The more standardized a procedure is, the more efficient and profitable it is. If we can see a higher number of pets and figure a common "recipe" or protocol to use on all similar cases, then more appointments can be accomplished.

Remember the universal business premise that time is money? Well, it's easy to understand how one of the most profitable areas in veterinary medicine is pharmaceuticals, Selling medicines, such as flea products and over the counter supplements, is usually a quick transaction that has a high return on investment with less costs to the clinic.

Perhaps TCVM has not taken off as quickly because it is not as efficient as selling products or as quick as, say, a vaccination appointment. It takes the holistic veterinarian additional personal time and funds to acquire the knowledge and then even more time to "reinvent the wheel" by treating each and every patient in a customized manner. Adding time to go over things that the owner can do at home to prevent disease can be considered non-income generating and time consuming practices.

Our profession should consider abandoning the human Health Maintenance Organization (HMO) model of practice, which maximizes the hours you work by doing high density appointment scheduling. Instead, one that invests more time with clients and patients would be a better health advocate for the pet parents. This novel approach of high quality time with clients versus quantity of appointments could offset the revenue loss of the HMO model by creating a better bond with clients. This formula also results in higher client loyalty and retention. Spending longer with the patient could result in finding other issues and thus generating more services. The "way things have always been done" is not a valid excuse nor the best way to practice.

Preventive medicine is our duty. I truly love helping sick pets heal, but I enjoy seeing healthy ones even more so. The "mechanistic" approach of modern medicine uses technology at all cost. Veterinary medicine has become very high tech as well, but in my opinion, it needs to also become "high touch". Alternative medicine relies on the practitioner's ability to use their hands, a comprehensive physical and emotional assessment of the pet, and an environmental assessment of the pet in order to diagnose. I happen to practice and support Integrative

Medicine, where some western diagnostic and treatments are used in conjunction with the TCVM and holistic approach. The answer is always balance in everything.

I was once presented a dog that had been seen by another clinic. The dog was acutely paralyzed and the owner was told if her pet did not have spinal surgery within twenty-four hours, it was at risk of never walking again. She was told that if she did not agree to the surgery that she should consider euthanasia.

The owner was very upset because she did not have $5,000 for the emergency spinal surgery. She posted her story on social media about what was happening. As luck will have it, one of my clients saw the post and sent her our way. The owner had never heard of alternative medicine or acupuncture for pets. We used an integrative approach using herbs, acupuncture, massage, muscle relaxants, and anti-inflammatories to manage her dog's case. To her happy surprise, he walked again within a few sessions.

We taught the owner how to perform massages at home to stimulate the bladder meridian and prevent future incidents. We prescribed a diet with a list of foods that supported the TCVM pattern that was given. The total cost of treatment was around $500 and the outcome was what we hoped for. If every emergency service would consider a referral for acupuncture and rehabilitation as an alternative to surgery, they could save many pets with owners that are not able to afford the higher costs of emergency back surgery.

The strength of allopathic medicine lies in the treatment of acute injuries and diseases, but what about chronic disorders? Most require frequent administration of drugs and blood monitoring to avoid side effects from the same medicines. A good example is the management of Cushing's disease, an adrenal gland related disorder. The common treatment is Vetoryl which is an expensive medication. All pets receiving this medication must have regular blood tests. One major side effect is inducing a fatal adrenal crisis from overmedication. Cushing's can be managed with a much safer herbal formula called Ophiopogon and regular acupuncture treatments. The cost of treatment is significantly less and the pet's health is less at risk. It may not work as a sole treatment in all cases, but if done in conjunction with Vetoryl, the chances of controlling this devastating disease improve considerably. As a bonus, a lower dose and frequency of drugs can be used, which in turn will limit the occurrence of damaging side effects.

I hope I made my case for Integrative Medicine being the best of both worlds. After all, if we put our patients' well-being first, we should use all the available tools to promote their healing.

CHAPTER 2

VACCINATION DEBATE

• • • •

To vaccinate or not to vaccinate your pet. This issue has brought up a lot of debate in the veterinary medical profession and caused great concerns for dedicated pet owners. In the human arena, there is a lot of activism against vaccinations. This movement has now spilled over into the pet world.

A debate broke out. On one side were celebrities who were touting that vaccinations cause children to have autism. They claimed that something within the vaccinations changed their children's mind forever.

On the other side of the argument were allopathic medicine practitioners, warning that by not vaccinating your child, you were not only putting your own child at risk, but every other child they came into contact with. Medical professionals painted a picture of apocalyptic proportions.

The result of the confusion has been that people do not know what to do. They want to protect their child on hand, but they do not want to hurt them in the process. Schools require a child to be vaccinated before they are allowed to attend. Even after the basic vaccinations, a school board could require more booster vaccinations during a serious outbreak of a disease, such as meningitis.

I don't treat humans and, even though I would like to avoid the debate, it has affected the decision making ability of pet owners. They want to protect their babies, but don't want to hurt them in the process.

The question remains the same whether you are talking about human babies or furry ones. Do you vaccinate or not vaccinate?

In reference to your pet, my answer is that it depends. There are so many factors affecting the decision on whether a vaccine is safe or recommended for your pet. It has to be considered on a case by case basis. It makes sense to me that a little dog that is basically aerial, never touches the floor, has a different need for protection than a hunting dog that lives in an outdoor kennel. To better understand the difference, you must first understand why we need vaccinations in the first place.

Vaccines challenge your pet's immune system to create antibodies to fight off a particular disease. Each vaccine contains an antigen, or an inactive disease causing organism. It does not need to be an entire micro-organism; it can merely be a piece of virus or bacteria. When we vaccinate our pets, their immune system becomes activated and creates antibodies specifically designed to kill that organism. It replicates those antibodies and places them into your pet's immunity arsenal. The next time the organism enters the body, the blueprint of the antibody is activated and your pet is able to fight the intruder.

Immune system activation is not a simple process.; it takes a lot of energy. A dog that is old, sick, weak, or otherwise compromised can become overtaxed, feeble, and even more susceptible to other diseases.

You might think there is just one vaccine for one disease, but there are number of companies that make their own version of a vaccine. If you want Ibuprofen, you not only have Advil brand to choose from, but nearly every store has their own brand. Even name brand prescriptions have generic equivalents.

Many people think that all of these equivalent medications are the same as the name brand, but that is not true. In fact, legally they cannot be the exact same compounds. They can be quite close, but they may have different inert ingredients, or the chemical compound has slightly been altered.

Not all vaccines are created equal either. There are a number of different companies all touting how their process creates the best and safest vaccine. Instead of a differing compound, vaccines are differentiated by the process used to create them. Some vaccines are considered killed, which means they contain whole dead organisms or parts of them in a solution. Others are labelled modified-live ones (MLV), which means they contain genetic codes bodies will use to create antibodies, but the organisms themselves have been rendered harmless.

So which kind of vaccine is better? Which one is safer? It depends on the health of your pet, what the vaccine is for, and why you are considering it. Most of the time when you take your pet in for a vaccination, they will not tell you what kind of vaccine they are administering, but you can always ask. You can even ask ahead and do some research on the brand they use in your vet's clinic. You are an advocate for your pet, and you do have choices about their health and well-being.

The modified live vaccines or MLVs are supposed to get better and longer immunity with fewer allergic reactions. MLVs do contain a modified disease-causing virus or bacteria that, in some pets, can cause a lesser form of the disease to actually manifest. Many people have this experience with Flu shots, which is a vaccination against the strain of Influenza the medical community feels is going to be the most common in a particular year. After receiving my last Flu shot, I became very sick with flu-like symptoms. It was not the actual flu, but to me it did not matter because I was still sick.

Since that experience, I have decided to focus on strengthening my immune system rather than risk the side effects of another shot. This type of reaction can happen in pets too. Some puppies will test positive for parvovirus after a MLV vaccine, and may suffer from adverse reactions like bloody stools and becoming ill.

Sometimes humans cannot tolerate generic brands of their medications, and usually the culprits are the inert ingredients. These are substances added to the medicine, but do not have medicinal properties. In pet vaccines, when a dead virus is used, an adjuvant is added. An adjuvant is a substance added to be an immune stimulator; it helps the immune system respond to the dead virus.

CORE VACCINES

Core vaccines are those widely recommended for all pets since they are common diseases. While these are recommended, I consider the age, health status, and lifestyle to be main determinants of whether a particular pet needs vaccinations or not.

Here is a list of what I refer to as blanket wall core vaccines. These are the ones most cats and dogs should have and that provide good protection.

Dogs:

» Canine adenovirus (CAV)

» Canine parvovirus (CPV)

» Canine distemper virus (CDV)

» Rabies

Cats:

» Feline herpesvirus 1 (FHV 1)

» Feline calicivirus (FCV)

» Feline panleukopenia virus (FPV)

» Rabies

All puppies and kitties under sixteen weeks should get three doses of the Core Vaccines as a MLV once every three weeks, then get the rabies vaccine. For dogs and cats older than sixteen weeks, they will need to be repeated at least twice if it is first time being immunized. There are products approved for three year durations and I recommend those for the second year booster vaccination.

Rabies vaccination schedules are determined by state laws and each state differs in regards to the minimal age that pets need to be vaccinated. At our practice we follow the Florida law that requires the dogs or cats to be at least twelve weeks of age.An initial vaccination followed by a yearly booster is advised and at the second yearly booster, our state allows the three-year rabies vaccine to be given.

NON-CORE VACCINES

There are other optional vaccines, referred to as Non-Core vaccines, which are often given because of a pet's geographic location. If you have ever travelled overseas, you are familiar with all of extra vaccinations you need before travelling for diseases such as Malaria and Typhoid. There are standard ones that are recommended for travel to certain countries and an additional list of vaccines depending on your health.

Your pets have the same kind of geographic health risks. Ask your veterinarian what Non-Core diseases are prevalent in your geographical area, are more common regarding your pet's lifestyle, and the degree of risk. A great example is the Lyme disease, which is more prevalent in the north-eastern states than compared with southern states. If a particular disease is common in your state or community, it should be considered an essential part of your pet's vaccine schedule.**Controversial Vaccines**

There are some lesser known vaccines which are controversial. The Feline Peritonitis (FIP) vaccine is one I have a personal aversion to, as I blame it on the death of my beloved cat-son Braulio. In 1990-1994, while in vet school, I adopted a Himalayan mix kitten who became my best friend and confidant. He was my emotional support and got me through the stress of moving to a foreign place, facing a tough graduate school in a different language, and losing my darling mother in my third year of Vet School.

As a student, we had low-cost services including vaccinations, and I was told to vaccinate him for FIP, which I did, even though I understood very little about the risks. I never questioned the small animal clinician recommendations and I vaccinated my cat, who was a totally indoor cat, for four years in a row.

It was only later, after my first job as a cat only practitioner, that I learned that the vaccine was really ineffective to prevent the deadly disease and that indoor cats were at a very low risk of contracting it. When my beloved friend fell ill with fluid in the lungs in 1997, the last thing on earth I thought caused it was FIP. When the pathologist's report was released, I called and asked how a completely healthy, indoor cat could contract this disease. The first question he asked was, "Did you vaccinate him?"

I was devastated and guilt ridden. The thought that, while trying to protect my sweet friend, I had caused his horrible death was unfathomable. The fact that this personal loss has influenced my views on vaccination is an understatement.

Another example of a lesser known vaccine is the Pythiosis vaccine, which fights against a deadly algae-like organism that lives in lakes. I happen to practice in the "city of lakes", with 144 of those bodies of water, and all or most contain this organism. The vaccine has lots of critics and is the center of many heated debates in academia.

Some local vets vaccinate regularly for it. I do not use it as a vaccine, but rather use it as a treatment for Pythiosis, and quite successfully. I remember a standard poodle named Bolt that had lost a lot of weight and kept vomiting despite aggressive allopathic treatment. After the owner told me he chewed sticks and mulch, I asked if she used lake water. When she said yes, I knew it was Pythiosis. I then took a blood sample and sent it stat and, unfortunately, was not surprised that it came positive. I vaccinated him with a series of three doses and, thankfully, it worked! Of course, the challenge in diagnosing Pythiosis is that it appears like many other gastric issues so by the time we test for it, it is often too late. If your dog swims and plays in a lake or if you use lake or well-water for your landscape, you should at least be aware of the risk Pythiosis and of life-saving treatments available. Knowledge is power, so ask your veterinarian about this or any vaccination, and push hard for reasons why they would recommend or not recommend using it.

Another disease affecting pond and lake-loving dogs is Leptospirosis. The bacteria that causes this disease has several strains and the vaccines available cover the four most common ones. Transmission of the bacteria is through infected urine from wildlife, especially rodents. What makes it a threat is that Leptospira bacteria can live in soil, ponds, and bodies of water for months! Therefore, dogs and cats that live or spend a lot of time outdoors, especially hunting dogs, are at risk to get this disease. Unfortunately, the symptoms of affected dogs are widely varied and this disease goes undiagnosed most of the time. If an outdoorsy pet suddenly stops eating, vomits, has a fever or is very weak, he needs to be taken to the veterinarian and tested for Leptospirosis. The main concerns are that this disease can cause fatal kidney and/or liver failure pretty quickly. If diagnosed at an early stage, the kidney and liver failure can be reversed with appropriate antibiotics.

The controversy and the reason many veterinarians do not vaccinate for this disease is because the carrier of that vaccine is associated with many adverse reactions, including anaphylaxis. The culprit on most of the cases of anaphylaxis I see is the Leptospirosis vaccine. One particular case I treated came to me as a second opinion due to a severe adverse reaction to that vaccine. Right after he received the vaccination he became paralyzed! The owner had originally refused the vaccination, but the veterinarian insisted that her mostly indoors dog could acquire the disease in their backyard. In Florida, our abundant wildlife makes every yard a potential threat so the veterinarian had a good argument. However, this dog had previously reacted to vaccines and had never been vaccinated with that specific bacteria. Luckily, this dog responded to the TCVM approach and recovered. Needless to say, I gave a vaccination exemption letter and lots of information to his owner on titers.In an "at risk" dog, the Leptospirosis vaccine benefit might override reaction concerns. This disease can affect humans too so, depending on the lifestyle of your dog, this vaccine could be considered a core one.

There is a balance. When the right vaccine is used in the right circumstances, they can be life-saving. I don't want to give the impression that I am "anti-vaccine" because I am not. What I do believe is that pet owners should be educated in order to make informed choices. I have seen extreme views on anti-vaccine agenda be harmful as well. If you refuse to vaccinate a healthy puppy that has been checked out and could receive one with minimal risk, then I think you are truly neglecting that pet.

I had a woman come in with a twelve week old puppy that was suffering with vomiting and diarrhea. We immediately suspected Parvo virus, a hemorrhagic gastroenteritis that is often fatal and very expensive to treat. She argued that she did not vaccinate her because she read on the internet about the harmful effects of vaccines.

That owner was frantic to learn that this disease would've been totally avoided had she vaccinated with the core parvo vaccine at eight weeks and then repeated at eleven weeks. After almost a week of hospitalization, this lucky little puppy made it. The majority of others don't though. My advice is to have all puppies go through the recommended veterinary guidelines for vaccinations up to sixteen weeks UNLESS your puppy reacts to any of them. If they react badly with vomiting, hives, pain, swelling, hair loss at the site injection, or diarrhea that means the vaccine provoked an abnormal "excessive" immune response and I think that pet can be protected with less immunizations. That type of reaction warrants titers instead of just vaccinating.

In my practice, I try at least two sets of vaccines three weeks apart, then do titers to see if a vaccine is needed. I truly do not advocate continuing to give vaccines to animals that have reacted badly. Allergic reactions tend to become worse with each exposure. I interpret bad reactions as their body trying to telling us something, so it is important that we listen.

In the vaccine insert, it says that the product is intended to be used on *healthy* animals. This means if your pet is battling cancer or any other systemic illnesses, you should not vaccinate it. I take the temperature of my patients before I vaccinate, if they have a fever I do not administer it. Period! The exception might be a three-year Rabies vaccine to comply with the laws regulating animal vaccinations.

There are many well-meaning pet owners who think that vaccinating their pet means that they are taking good care of them. The vaccine clinics certainly promote this sentiment, but I would challenge that notion. Vaccines can sometimes be harmful for your pet. The only way to be sure you not taking unnecessary risks is to have your vet do a good physical exam and assessment to make a well-founded professional recommendation.

Vaccine safety, like other pharmaceuticals, operates in the realm of ranges. Each dog and cat breed has their own set of unique traits and characteristics. It is these differences that often enamor us to a particular breed. For instance, I absolutely love German Shepherds and Pugs, two polar opposites when it comes to traits and character.

German Shepherds are a large breed, hardy and intelligent, but they are also known to have GI and Arthritis issues.

Pugs, on the other hand, are flat-faced, small, pudgy, and super friendly breed with predisposed respiratory and heart issues. Now, think about this from a vet's position.

Why would I need to give the same dose of vaccine for these two very different beings? All veterinary drug dosages take into account the weight of the animal, but that is not true when it comes to vaccines. My greatest concern with this 'one size fits all dosing" is adverse reactions, especially when I am presented with teacup size breeds, 3lbs and under. I do not give multiple vaccines at once, if no adverse reactions present themselves, then I give the rest of the vaccines a week later. In addition, it is legal for veterinarians to split the dose of any vaccine except for Rabies.

If there are fears that the dose is not eliciting a good response, then a titer can be given several weeks later for peace of mind. I sometimes inject on GV14 (located midline on the back of the lower neck, as it meets the chest) which is an acupuncture point that stimulates the immune system on all animals.

Sometimes a vaccine is not effective the first time around or the effectiveness has waned over time. This is why we have yearly vaccines because the immunity for certain vaccines does not last forever. One of the ways to determine whether a pet needs a booster vaccine is to draw a titer. This is a blood test that shows whether the antibodies for a particular disease are present. If the response is strong, then your pet may not need another vaccine. As I have already mentioned, vaccines can really put a lot of pressure on your pet's immune system, so why over-vaccinate them if they don't need it?

I've even had littermates and housemates that have equal exposure to vaccines get vaccine titers and, surprisingly, one always ends up needing a booster. Why? Unlike robots, animals have individual characteristics that affect the level of immune response. Does it make any sense to treat them the same? Why not alter the frequency to suit their individual response to the immune challenge? On the other hand, if a known reactor's littermate comes for vaccines, I would be very conservative and will not give multiple vaccines on one visit. Most reactions happen seventy-two hours post vaccination so I advise owners to give Benadryl up to three days post vaccination to avoid a reaction. If your pet vomits, acts feverish, acts tired or very painful right after receiving a vaccine, it is considered having an adverse reaction. Sadly, early in my career, I had two pets die from anaphylaxis within twenty-four hours of having their vaccinations updated. Those deaths have influenced the way I practice and the vaccination protocols I have embraced since.

I try to never vaccinate incoming boarders the same day they come in, I prefer to vaccinate them two weeks prior to boarding. In a few cases, I've had to give them the day they leave. Why worry about timing? Mainly because stress is a big influence on the immune system and it can diminish an appropriate response. If you are boarding your pets, ask for the absolute minimal vaccine required and update at least two weeks prior to leaving them in. Alternatively, do a titer and bring that as proof of protection.

Another unsavory issue with over-vaccination is the possibility of the vaccine causing a soft tissue sarcoma, or a skin tumor. When I first started practicing at an all cat clinic twenty-two years ago, this was an emerging concern. I saw three cases of cats developing lumps at the site of vaccination. Unfortunately, in 1996 there were no general guidelines as to how to vaccinate pets.

After the second case, I talked to my boss, the late Dr. Alspach, about my concern that the vaccines could be causing the tumors. We were mixing the feline leukemia vaccine with all of the core feline vaccines and injected it all at once. After seeing these cases, we started separating them and using specific spots in the body for each of them long before it became standard practice in the rest of the veterinary community. These sarcoma tumors are very invasive, and even when removed, they would come back. Sadly, all three of those cats ended up having to be euthanized. I was devastated about it and those feelings of guilt have guided me to really weigh every recommendation I make to my clients. Even though I am very conservative and use the purest vaccines, on a rare few occasions, I've still seen fibro sarcomas after administering a vaccination. When these occur, I treat them with a TCVM protocol in combination with a wide surgical resection, using a laser, to treat them.

I had a case of a Siamese cat in which I treated for fibro sarcoma. She had three years of remission after my combined treatment. The second remission time, just under two years caused by other health issues, we put her to sleep. I have another case of a handsome big gray fluffy cat that has been on remission for over eight years after a fibro sarcoma related to a rabies vaccine. Of course, neither of these two patients ever got vaccinated again.What does risk assessment really mean? It is an analysis of you and your pet's lifestyle and the probability that such lifestyle will put your pet at risk of getting diseases. Lifestyle can vary so much; are you a frequent camper/traveler vs stationary, is your pet mainly indoors vs outdoors, do you walk your pet in public roads vs own backyard, is your pet an only child vs multiple pet/species in household?

This is key information that we use to determine if your pet is at risk of getting disease. We also consider the age of the pet, previous health issues, breed/species propensities, and even diet. I remember a beagle named Dixie, a rat hunter who occasionally ate rabbits. She was extremely healthy and fit. I had given her a Rabies vaccine at twelve years of age and exempted her from anymore vaccines due to age. When she was eighteen, she went to the emergency clinic having neurological signs and seizures. She was suspected of having a brain tumor and, since the Rabies was out of date, a Rabies suspect. The owner transferred her to us for the rabies quarantine. Just because I knew her preference to be outdoors and her ability to hunt small wildlife (bunnies, rats, moles), I thought she could have acquired Toxoplasmosis.

Infection with the parasite Toxoplasma Gondii causes neurological symptoms similar to Rabies, but it responds to treatment. These parasites can be transmitted by eating rodents, so I started treating her for it. I was pretty sure the Rabies vaccine titer would come in high since she had it all her life up to twelve years and it did. Although I did not submit the testing for Toxoplasmosis, I was confident it was the most likely cause of her symptoms. Sure enough, she made a full recovery within forty-eight hours of the new treatment and went on to live three more active years. I learned my lesson and now tell owners of hunting dogs to get the Rabies titer if their pet is still hunting, regardless of how old they are. Dixie proved to me that sometimes age is just a number.

A special consideration has to be given to small exotic pets. I love taking care of "pocket" pets (rats, mice, hamsters, etc.), reptiles, birds, and ferrets at my practice. Most do not need vaccines. I only vaccinate ferrets using a specific vaccine for ferret distemper and the Rabies three-year vaccine. Ferrets can scratch and bite, so for liability purposes I recommend the Rabies vaccine every year. Veterinarians cannot predict the vaccine protection in exotics as well as we can with dogs and cats, so I err on the side of caution. I tell my ferret owners to wait fifteen minutes post vaccination because, in my experience, ferrets will react to vaccines pretty quickly. They may start vomiting, have their pads turn red, and they go limp. In my experience, maybe 1 out of 10 ferrets react to the Distemper vaccine whereas about 1 in 25 will react to the Rabies. Production of the ferret Distemper vaccine has been discontinued several times and some veterinarians have used a canine distemper vaccine instead. I feel the ferret specific one was the safest option and do not advise using the canine counterpart.

Another common practice I do not condone is vaccinating at the time of spay or neuter. It is like telling an overworked horse to double its cargo. Let us think through this logically. Your pet is having a major surgery that will engage the immune system in healing, so why would you want to add more stress on top of it? Most of the time it is for nothing more than convenience. The animal is asleep and so it is easy to give them the vaccine and saves another trip to the office.

Sadly, most shelters and government run animal services vaccinate at same time of sterilization. Why? Shelter medicine is geared to adopt out in as short time as possible and, to do that, they do as much as they can at the same time. Luckily, your pets have the luxury of waiting for the optimal time to vaccinate.

My flexible vaccination approach may seem common sense with the evidence of studies proving that the immunity produced by certain vaccines can last from two to seven years! In fact, these studies were the reason vaccination guidelines came to exist. My profession realized we were just blindly following manufacturer's recommendations without testing if they were really needed. Most veterinarians take the oath of "Do No Harm" seriously and want to do what is best for your pet.

DECLINING A VACCINE

There are a lot of veterinarians and clinics around the US. According the AVMA, in 2014, there were an estimated 65,600 veterinarian practices in the U.S. You have choices. It is important that you are comfortable with your vet and that you share the same ideal of health and wellness for your pet.

The good news is that, as a pet owner, you can decline a vaccination anytime. Ask your veterinarian to evaluate the risk your pet's lifestyle has and then let him or her make a vaccine recommendation based on that. Your veterinarian might offer to sign a vaccination waiver that can be added to your pet's medical records.

It is your pet and your choice. You should get your puppies vaccinated, unless there is a reason not to, and boosters can be administered, but remember that titers are an acceptable option. You want to do the right thing and I want your pet to live a long and healthy life. My goal is to be sure to provide pet owners with solid information based upon medical studies and my professional experience. Involve your veterinarian and ask about the risk factors of vaccinating. Become educated about vaccinations, and do your due diligence before you take your pet in. It is your obligation as a pet owner to get the best and most appropriate care for your pet.

CHAPTER 3

ENERGETIC FIELD

• • • •

WE ARE ALL MADE UP OF ENERGY and that energy radiates beyond our bodies. This concept applies to animals and is known in the area of alternative medicine as the bio-field or morphogenetic fields. These fields are complex and include electromagnetic waves along with light emission properties. I regard the idea that our pets are wrapped in a cocoon of invisible energy field that contains information about their bodies as a valuable tool to assist me in helping to heal them.

Russian biologist Alexander Gurwitsch first proposed the theory of morphogenetic fields in the early 1900's. He believed that embryos received some external information that directed them in a specific sequence of development. In other words, there was a cohesive, organizing force outside of the cells that developed them into a specific organism.

Think that Gurwitsch idea is crazy? Remember that the technology that powers our cell phones communicates by transmitting radio waves and radio frequency waves are actually electromagnetic fields. The same way that cell phones create radio waves that transmit information through the air, pet cells are like mini cell phones constantly transmitting information.

Gurwitsch also discovered the bio-photon, which is a weak electromagnetic wave and light emission from an animal or plant cell. This bio-photon light is detected in the ultraviolet range of the spectrum. Since then, there have been several scientific studies that have proven that all living cells produce light, or photons. Of course, the amount of light produced is very low, but some scientists have proven that healthy organisms produce higher photons than sick ones. This discovery is important because light also carries information. It supports the theory that this bio-field has information carried in those electromagnetic waves to help keep organisms healthy.

The relevance of this concept to my practice is two-fold. First, if the energy and information expands beyond the physical body then, the modality of energy healing, without even touching the pet, is validated. Second, I believe there is an exchange of information between humans and their close pets at the level of these bio-fields. This accounts for the prevalence of the same diseases expressed in both owner and their pet and for the nonverbal communication that seems to be shared in closely bonded humans and their pets.

It was after a documentary on energy healing modalities that I learned about the bio-field and the way healers manipulate it to achieve positive changes in their patient's health. One of those modalities is called Reconnection and is taught by famous chiropractor Dr. Eric Pearl. In 2011, after I became certified in acupuncture courses and was seeing how energy traveled in orderly ways within our bodies, I came across Dr. Pearl's work. I was skeptical, but intrigued. I then attended a class and was instantly hooked on energy healing. I performed the Reconnection on my family members, though never with the intention to practice it in people, and my personal pets. Soon enough it became another tool to help me treat my animal patients.

When I examine a pet, I quickly scan the energetic field to know which areas need attention. For example, in any painful or paralyzed animal, I scan the spine using the palm of my hand while concentrating on any reaction interacting with the animal's field. When my palms receive a prickling sensation, that tells me there is a disturbance to the energy flow. Then I use my hands to palpate the area and see if I elicit pain, then take radiographs. I find that radiographic evidence correlates to the troubled scanned area around 85% of the time!

In cases where the bloodwork and x-rays have failed to pinpoint a source of discomfort for the pet, I try to scan and focus on detecting any areas of disruption of the body's bio field.

The first law, also known as Law of Conservation of Energy, states that energy cannot be created or destroyed in an isolated system. The second law of thermodynamics states that the entropy of any isolated system always increases.

Our bodies and our pet's bodies are isolated systems. We eat and take that energy to move, and talk, and bark. But once that energy is used where does it go? It cannot be destroyed. What does energy look like in food? Can you see it? What does it look like in our bodies? We can't see that either.

We rely on instruments like an EKG or an EEG to pick up energy patterns from our bodies. Our bodies are bioelectric. It is this bioelectricity that allows us to move, feel, and digest food. It is the energy that allows you to convert light into sight. Once it is used in the body, where does it go?

An EEG picks up electrical impulses from our brains and translates them to a pen that moves and scratches. It is recording energy that is being released by the body. An EKG does something similar but it is recording the electrical impulses of your beating heart.

We have figured out that certain squiggles mean certain things, like a heart attack or a seizure.

We use little electrical detection devices on the body that can sense these energy patterns. It could seem like voodoo to someone who does not understand modern science. We have accepted that these devices work and that we can interpret the energy signals from the body. Why then, is it such a stretch to think we cannot also sense them with our hands?

Acupuncture explains the Meridians as the channels of organized energy travelling through the pet's body. What I am trying to propose here is that this energy extends further out, takes on an electromagnetic wave pattern, and might not be limited by the boundary imposed by our pet's flesh.

Skeptics may point out there haven't been any published scientific studies to prove that a person can detect an energy field. There haven't been studies that conclusively disprove it either. In addition, this field of energy medicine is facing many financial challenges curtailing the ability to produce more research and scientific studies. I expect that as these challenges are met, more data will validate the thousands of testimonials out there claiming healings by some form of energy medicine.

As a seasoned veterinarian, I can tell you that cats seem to have uncanny access to the energetic fields of their human staff. The bulk of all re-scheduled and missed feline appointments at my practice are due to the inability of cat owners to find their precious kitties come time for their appointments. Some critics will say that the cats are simply observant and they pick up cues from their owners' behaviors or changes in routine, like getting the cat carriers out. They may be partially right, but there are cases when the owners do not change routine on purpose. They try to sneak on their napping kitties with a classic grab-and-dunk in the carrier maneuver, only to be foiled by a hyper alert furry specter dashing under the bed or some unreachable bolt hole inside of the house. I find the explanation of an information exchange of the owner and cat body fields to be an elegant hypothesis that can explain this legendary cat behavior mystery.

Another common occurrence is that pets seem to know when the owners are coming home, even when they are far enough that they could not possibly sense it. Are pets psychic or is a sixth sense at play? Could the bio field information expand way further than what we imagine? This phenomenon has been studied by British biologist Rupert Sheldrake. He demonstrated statistical significant results that prove that there is some anticipatory behavior that cannot be explained by normal sensory perception or behavioral cues.

In his famous experiment, he videotaped an owner and her dog for a month. The owner was instructed to come home at different times and through different ways of transportation (bicycle, car, bus, walking). The dog went to the window next to the door in anticipation of his owner's arrival 24 out of 30 days. The six times that he did not go to the window corresponded to the dog being sick or was the day after an extensive walking or playing session.

Regardless of the method of transport or time of arrival, the dog impressively moved in position the second the owner started in the direction to the apartment. The study proved the dog anticipatory behavior was right a whopping 80% of the time, which is far greater than the 50/50 expected chance.

The theory of a bio field also explains a common phenomenon we observe at our practice, where pets and owners sharing the same disease process. I have several diabetic patients that have diabetic dogs and cats. One might think that perhaps lifestyle or environment might be affecting both humans and pets alike. However, I get to see too many coincidences including specific cancers (lymphoma, breast cancer), seizures, thyroid issues and organ failure affecting pet and owner in same household.

Take for example the story of a dear client suffering from breast cancer. When I told her that her dog had a suspicious lump in her breast that I needed to take out, she started to cry. She explained how she was battling breast cancer and had lost her aunt to it as well. She asked me if she somehow gave it to her dog. I assured her breast cancer wasn't contagious and that perhaps there were environmental pollution factors at play since those could affect both humans and pets.

However, I admit to have been pensive about that "coincidence" and started asking my clients that were being diagnosed with cancer, low thyroid, and diabetes if they or someone in the household had suffered a similar condition. To my surprise, a pattern of people sharing their pet's ailment emerged. The incidence was definitively higher than the 50/50 chance and included less common ailments as IBD, previous fractures, and same joint arthritis.

In one case, this inquiry process became a lifesaver! The dog had chronic skin and ear problems. I convinced the owner to invest in allergy testing and the results proved that her dog was allergic to mold. The owner had been feeling tired and had low energy and asked me if it was possibly related. I told her that her dog was reacting to something inside the house. She called some professionals and sure enough, they found black mold in her house! After her insurance replaced all the walls and the leaky plumbing that caused the mold, both her and her dog's symptoms disappeared.

In some cultures, pets serve as shields against evil. I happen to think that they are the canaries in the coal mine, telling us to pay attention to the quality of our environments and to take better care of ourselves.

Many pet owners tell me that they know what their pet is thinking or feeling and that their pet seems to anticipate their moods and actions. Most veterinarians agree that there are certain breeds of dogs (Dachshunds) and cats (Siamese) that seem to bond closely with just one human. My experience involves my cat Saatchi, who I got as a tiny kitten when I was a thirteen-year old and shared everything with her, including my bed. She did not care to pay attention to anyone, but me. I took her to college in Puerto Rico and she was the best roommate. She was extremely in tune with me, anticipated my arrivals, and seemed to know my moods. I loved her deeply. When I was accepted to Tuskegee University Veterinary School, I was a twenty-year old naive girl travelling with 200 dollars and no clear way on a housing option. My mother asked me to leave Saatchi behind and to collect her when I came back in the December break. I was heartbroken, but the reality of my precarious situation set in, so I relented.

Saatchi was extremely affectionate and clingy right before I left her, but when I came back for her in December she could not stand to be in the same room with me! She hissed at me and wanted nothing to do with me. I discovered that she had been refusing to eat and meowing a lot when I left and my mother started to allow her to sleep in her bed. My mom was sick with Hepatitis and Saatchi became her devoted companion. Right before my mother passed, Saatchi started to act strange and leaving the house more often. We suspect she was hit by a car, as she had disappeared.

Her behavior demonstrated to me the depth of emotion that cats, and animals in general, are capable of and that they mysteriously form special bonds with their pet owners. It also showed Siamese have good memory since she did not forgive me in the three years after that incident. That's why I think having a pet is a great responsibility. Millions of abandoned pets suffer the betrayal of their owners and are scarred emotionally. Luckily, pets have a tremendous ability to form deep bonds and live in the moment, which helps them adapt to new relationships with humans.

I truly believe that the bond between humans and their beloved pets goes deeper than we suspect, right at the quantum level.

CHAPTER 4

HEALING WITH INTENTION

• • • •

I N MY OPINION, THE SUCCESSFULNESS of a treatment depends of multiple factors. The animal's state of health, personality, stress, environmental conditions, dietary support, experience of the doctor and attitude of both doctor and the owner contribute to the treatment's success. Some people might question why I would say attitude can affect the outcome of the treatment. This reasoning is based on the proven fact that our thinking can affect the results of treatments—it is called the Placebo effect. This placebo means that just by believing that the treatment is effective, despite being a null treatment, the patient will experience healing. Of course, just like the *Yin* and the *Yang*, there is a counter effect called the Nocebo.The concept of the placebo effect has been around since the 1950's and has been a subject of study and controversy since. Several published papers proved that the placebo effect is directly responsible for 35% of all healings. In the article "The Placebo Prescription" by Margaret Talbot (*New York Times Magazine*, January 9, 2000) the author provides a compilation of examples of placebo experiments. Most impressive to many, is a study in which researchers told asthmatics that they were inhaling bronchodilators and it resulted in dilation of their airways. Can you imagine the biochemical reactions that needed to take place for the airways to enlarge? It is amazing to me that the sheer belief they were getting medicine actually caused a physical and measurable change in their bodies.

How can the placebo effect be important for healing our pets? The first thing we have to learn is the placebo doesn't directly apply to the pets because dogs and cats lack self-awareness. However, the same way the placebo explains how our mental state can potentiate healing is the way I understand to help our pets. If you decrease stressful situations around sick animals and instead surround them with a sense of safety, connection, and a positive environment, you increase the odds of that pet's recovery. Since you are the caregiver and have a close bond with your pet, your state of mind is directly influencing your dear pet's mind as well.

The veterinarian's belief in the efficacy of their treatment and on the prognosis of that disease will also play a major role in your pet's healing as well. I remember going to a lecture on a hard to treat disease called Autoimmune Hemolytic Anemia (AIHA) and being dismayed about the speaker's conclusion that it had a very high fatality rate. I reflected that in my first fifteen years I had never lost a patient to it and believed that it was a matter of treating promptly and thoroughly to successfully treat the majority of the cases. I turned around and looked at a colleague that worked at a nearby emergency clinic and said, "Can you believe that? He must be polling from flawed data, there is no way this has such a high mortality rate." Imagine my shock when she said they saw the same fatality rates or even higher at their clinic. Within a couple of weeks after I came back from the conference, I had a case of AIHA and, armed with the new protocols I had just learned, I treated the poor pet. Sadly, despite my treatment, the pet died. Then, thanks to Murphy's law (and the law that says problems come in three's), I had a second and third case all within a month!

I immediately worked hard on the second case. It looked like they would recover, but quickly relapsed and the owner elected for euthanasia. It dawned on me that my belief in the disease process was affecting my results. I had a mental conversation with myself and did some deep reflection on past cases and thought about those treatments. I was mentally prepared for that third case and was relieved when she made it through without relapse. Was I having a Nocebo effect on my treatment? Were my negative thoughts and outlook impacting the healing process? I can't be 100% certain, but I know that the whole experience affected how I look at any disease process ever since. The only thing I know for sure is that my clients and their pets can relax knowing they have an optimist as their doctor.

I remember what my good friend and client retired anesthesiologist Dr. Nagel said to me when I told him that his geriatric kitty's painful hips were due to degenerative joint disease and that I could do acupuncture to ease his pain. Dr. Nagel looked me in the eyes and proclaimed, "I think Acupuncture is rubbish and just a Placebo. I don't believe in it". I held his gaze and answered, "Great! Your kitty doesn't believe in it either! It is enough that I believe and am confident it will help your cat!". His cat responded marvelously and lived several pain free years afterwards. Until this day he tells me that he still doesn't believe in acupuncture, but he believes in me.

Throughout this book I have exhorted all pet owners to ask their veterinarians' input and to form a collaborative relationship with regards to the health decisions affecting your pet. Having a positive-minded veterinarian in your corner can be a great advantage when it comes to their handling of your pet's illnesses. Keeping hysterics at bay and focusing on obtaining a favorable outcome is your duty as a pet owner. Remember that your pet can sense your calm and assertive attitude, which will in turn make your pet more calm and submissive.

Growing up Catholic, and as superstitious as any other Puerto Rican, means I'm very open to the spiritual and unexplained realms of life. I believe that prayer is basically using intention to achieve results.

Whether you believe in the existence of God or a higher power or not, you can admit there are unexplained miracles of healing every day. I am not ashamed to say that I pray over my patients and their owners all the time. I actually ask the two prayer communities I belong to on social media to pray for specific cases too. I would venture to say that most of those critical cases do experience positive outcomes.

How can praying or deeply meditating on your pet's illness actually help them recover? There are many scientific papers trying to find the actual mechanism of intention healing and prayers. There are institutions like the National Institute of Health dedicating parts of its budget to fund studies to prove or disprove these alternative healing modalities. I can tell you that there are three main ways that most serious scientists try to explain prayer; that prayer or intention healing is a form of meditation, that it is a way to engage the placebo effect, or that prayer is coincidental with spontaneous remissions of the diseases.

I agree with the premise that prayer or intention healing is a form of meditation. The practice of meditation has been scientifically proven to have many benefits including decreasing stress, improving focus, and boosting the immune response. It makes sense that when a person prays or focuses on a particular pet, they are entering a meditative like trance that can benefit themselves. How can it travel out towards the intended pet though? I think the answer lies in our understanding that thoughts are a form of energy according to many scientists and quantum physicists. As mentioned in previous chapters, our universe is an energetic soup vibrating at different speeds and our body's energy is not contained within the barriers of our skin. Thoughts are emissions of energy and, as we said before, energy carries information. Assuming this is true then, prayer or intention is a thought or series of thoughts vibrating at a healing speed and focused on a specific target.

"The atoms of our bodies are traceable to stars that manufactured them in their cores and exploded these enriched ingredients across our galaxy, billions of years ago. For this reason, we are biologically connected to every other living thing in the world. We are chemically connected to all molecules on Earth. And we are atomically connected to all atoms in the universe. We are not figuratively, but literally stardust."

—Neil deGrasse Tyson

Think about the power of thoughts for a minute and it becomes clear that it is better for our health and for that of our pets to have a positive outlook in life. Experiments in quantum physics have shown that observing an electron, a small unit of energy, can change its behavior. If the electron was observed it behaved as a particle, but when it was not, it behaved as a wave. In other words, when we focus our attention and thoughts on something, we affect it.

Remember that your pet looks up to you and to all the cues we give them about our moods then behave accordingly. The opposite is true, their behavior effects our moods. It is scientifically proven that petting a dog or cat lowers our blood pressure and decreases our stress. These responses have profound effects on our neurochemistry and biology. It makes sense to think that conversely, if we obsessively fix our thoughts on the worst outcomes, we could slow down our pet's healing process.

At my animal hospital, we strive to decrease stress in all handling of our pets. We have attained certifications for hospital wide training in feline low stress handling techniques. We also have an animal behaviorist on staff, ready to address problems behaviors and give positive reward training to both pet owners and their dogs. My staff understands my prime directive: we must approach all animals with the intention of a quick, safe, and productive visit.

I also talk to the cats or dogs that I am treating and state my intention verbally and, more importantly, with my thoughts. Many clients have complimented me on my "pet manners". They laugh when I call their female pets "mama linda",pretty mommy, or their males "papa lindo", pretty pop,. What they don't hear is the mantra I am mentally repeating, "I am your friend, I want to help you, let me help you, thank you for letting me help you". Also, I strongly visualize the pet cooperating and try to imagine how the problem will look already solved.

I have been nicknamed "the cat whisperer" by my staff and on several occasions I've been asked by clients if I was a trained animal communicator. When I first heard the term animal communicator, I thought that it was a ridiculous notion and a scam. However, I've had multiple clients who have consulted animal communicators with enough success to make me curious. So, I researched the topic and learned their techniques were very similar to what I was doing intuitively. They basically send mental images and loving thoughts towards the pet, which to me means using the power of intention. The difference is that they claim to receive mental images back and can piece together a story of what is happening with that pet. I'm definitely a one-way communicator then!

Intention can be a very useful tool for practitioners and technicians alike. For example, when I need to collect blood and attempt hitting a vein or need to place an intravenous catheter, I rarely miss. Why? I first ask permission to the pet. Then I visualize the vein before I attempt the draw and I send loving, peaceful thoughts to that pet. I taught my technicians to do the same and it has made a great impact in the efficiency of my staff.

Originally there were doubters who thought that I was making this concept up. However, they could not deny the evidence for long. They witnessed how I would approach pets that were trying to attack them or being difficult, but in an instant behaved calmly with me. Interestingly, most of my new clients with famously aggressive pets are also surprised to see their babies behaving differently, more calmed, relax and cooperative, at our clinic.

My whole staff has bought into the concept of intention healing. Our goal is to make every interaction with our pet patients a positive experience so that when these pets return to visit us, they are at ease and unafraid.

My team has found nice ways of conveying love and compassion to the pets under our care. For example, we routinely hug our pet patients after surgical procedures. We wrap the pets in a nice comfy blanket, hold them, and talk soothingly until they are more conscious over the trembling and dissociative mental state that happens while recovering from the anesthesia. This results in smoother awakenings and avoids any trauma associated with us. In addition, we cover the sick pets' cages with scented calming pheromones, or chemical scents produced by the pet's bodies that elicit good feelings as response, use soothing music, or turn the lights off in order to put them at ease.

Our whole team offers positive conditioning using petting or treats for all procedures. The dogs boarding at our deluxe boarding have the dog-specific channel Dog TV playing ten hours a day in their rooms. The cat boarding room is sound proofed to avoid stress from hearing dogs barking and constantly plays a music CD created to soothe cats. We make sure our side of the healing equation is fulfilled by providing positive-minded doctors and veterinary nurses along with the low stress, loving environment.

I felt that our efforts to be a safe haven for pets were paying off when, during an afternoon storm, a rambunctious yellow lab with storm anxiety showed up at the hospital's front door demanding entrance. He escaped his own yard to come be safe with us!

A black Cocker Spaniel named Ms. Maggie Lee is another great example of a happily conditioned pet. She puts on a happy display and pulls the owner into the hospital for her weekly daycare and spa day. She adores the kennel staff and doesn't even need to be walked on a leash. She knows exactly where she is going and can't wait to be there.

We still miss our sweet friend Sasha, an Alaskan Malamute, that came for morning daycare Monday to Friday for over a decade! Not only did she look forward to visiting our practice and enjoying playtime with other dogs, but the owner once told me she would "pout' in the rare occasions when she had to stay home. Many of our clients tell us that they can sense their pets love coming to us. The few that are nervous or hesitant to come in still behave pretty well.

Another confirmation we were doing a good job was when we were being audited by our Worker's Compensation firm. The representative commented that she had never seen a hospital with almost zero claims concerning animal bites or scratches. I wonder what she would have said if I told her that our secret was a combination of treats and affection.

I consider myself an intuitive healer, which means I listen to my "gut" when I am treating or diagnosing animals. I also listen to the owners and ask how they feel about my recommendations because if they are having negative thoughts about the procedures I suggested, they can influence the outcome.

A good example is the story of Sheena, a twelve year old dog that had a "benign" fatty lump, lipoma, on her chest. This tumor had progressively grown so large that it was in danger of outrunning its blood supply. All tumors create new blood vessels, angiogenesis, to feed themselves. When they grow faster than their blood supply, the core of the tumor mass starts to die. After the core dies, the tumor mass ruptures and nasty decayed tumor flesh is exposed. In some cases, veins and arteries are also exposed and the animal is in danger of losing a lot of blood. If the tumor is in the skin, like Sheeba's was, it's marginally better than a tumor mass inside the abdomen, like the spleen or liver. With skin tumors bursting at least you can notice it and bandage or surgically remove it. Regardless, it is a situation that both pet owner and veterinarian prefer to avoid.

The owner was very concerned and told me that she had a feeling her dog could not go through anesthesia. I assuaged all her fears by telling her that her pet's pre-surgical bloodwork and heart were looking well and that it was a simple surgery, not to last longer than a half hour. The day of the surgery came. As I was about to start cutting the skin, the dog stopped breathing. Her heart slowed down enough to concern me and I started CPR and breathing for her with the Ambu-bag. I watched the clock to keep time of contractions and put the incident in her notes. I noted the time around ten o'clock in the morning. After five minutes, we finally got her back to being stable and I quickly finished the surgery. It was around noon after she recovered and was up and around. I soon called the owner. Her voice was trembling when she answered. She confessed that she was afraid that I called to say her dog had died. I was surprised and asked why she thought the worst. At precisely at ten in the morning, she was at her work desk and felt the presence of her dog pressing on her leg. She felt a deep love and peace feeling overcoming her. I was in shock and still to this day wonder if that dog's spirit went to her owner.

After that day, I decided if the owner has a strong opposition against a procedure, was not willing to take ANY risks, or that I cannot completely reassure them with all my precautions against an adverse event, then I won't do the procedure at all.

Intention healing is another tool in my treatment toolbox. Skeptics might question its effectiveness, but I get to see the day to day successful outcomes of using a positive, mindful attitude towards each pet patient. It has also made me very in tune with the pet owners and improved my communication skills greatly. As a bonus, I get to enjoy working in a nurturing and caring environment, where work almost feel like play.

CHAPTER 5

HEALING WITH ACUPUNCTURE

• • • •

THE MOST COMMON QUESTION asked about acupuncture is how does it work? I'll try to answer that by explaining what are those special acupoints in the body are, how can we stimulate them, and when is it appropriate to do so.

Interestingly, acupuncture points were identified by the Chinese several millennia ago. The undeniable fact is if these points are stimulated, there will be a physiological response. Needles of different sizes and materials are used, but are usually painless or at least less painful than needles used for injections. Proficient practitioners use their hands to feel the acupuncture point; they do not rely on just anatomical descriptions.

Any pressure on that acupoint will result in stimulation. Therefore, we could use our fingers, we could inject liquids or air under the skin surface above the point, or we could bleed out the specific acupoints. Even when we come to the decision to use needles to hit the acupoint, we have many choices; apply heat, connect to electricity, or just use a simple "dry" needle.

Modern research shows that acupoints are located in areas where there is a high density of free nerve endings, mast cells, arteries, and lymphatic vessels. Most of these acupoints are motor points, which means there is a nerve that makes a specific part of the body move. A lot of the studies made by National Institutes of Health and the World Health Organization also indicate that stimulation to these special points results in endorphins, serotonin, and other neurotransmitters released. Skeptical pet owners would be surprised to know that there are over 20,000 articles regarding acupuncture effects.

There are three main scientifically proven ways that can explain the physiological effects of acupuncture. First, acupoints have been found to be conductors of electromagnetic signals. When an acupoint is stimulated with a needle, the signals increase along the pathway and stimulate the central nervous system (CNS). This will then release the flow of pain killing endorphins and immune system cells that aid in healing. These electromagnetic signals can be measured and shows how points could be found using modern devices that detect those signals.

Have you ever had a light go out in your home and thought it was just burned out? You touch it to unscrew it and it flickers. You realize that the problem is not the bulb, but the connection. We diagnose diseases in Western medicine like we have a broken bulb. If we can't fix it with medication, we remove it or, in some cases replace it, like surgery. Acupuncture is effective in fixing the flow of energy. Sometimes the bulb is burned out and needs more invasive action, but acupuncture can heal many problems without the need of more intense Western Medicine intervention.

The second method of action is by activating the Opioid system, which tells the brain to release chemicals that ease pain into the CNS. These are the body's own literal drug store.

Third, the acupuncture stimulation directly alters the brain chemistry by releasing neurotransmitters and neurohormones that control the body's blood pressure, blood flow, body temperature, and promote sensations of wellbeing.

Modern medicine is now reaching out to integrate the wisdom of acupuncture into treatments. For example, that little stripe of tape that athletes use in the middle of their nose to breathe better or as a way to stop snoring is actually stimulating a specific acupuncture point known to open the sinuses called *Bi tong*. How about the device in the lower back that is used to help people with urinary incontinence? Many women that have had an ovarian hysterectomy or men that had prostate surgery, end up having difficulty with urinary incontinence. They choose to have an implant in their lower back to correct the issue. This is achieved by sacral nerve stimulation (SNS) using an electrical stimulator under the person's skin above their buttocks. Electrodes are attached to it to send pulses to the sacral nerve in the lower back. Well, this implant is stimulating classical acupoints called *Shen Shu* and an acupoint called Bladder 28, which are the acupoints specific for toning kidney and bladder! The energy goes into the nerves that supply the bladder and helps the sphincter hold on. This issue is also one of the causes of urinary incontinence in dogs and cats.

Urinary incontinence is a very common issue in aging pets, especially female dogs and cats that are spayed under three months of age. There appears to be very little that western intervention can do about this issue, other than ruling out incontinence caused by kidney or bladder diseases, urinary stones, cancer or congenital deformations of the urinary tracts using diagnostics like bloodwork, xrays, bacterial cultures, etc. Of course, if an underlying reason is not found, the treatment involves life-long medications. Sadly, many pets end up being euthanized because the owners cannot deal with this issue. Although a SNS implant is not available for dogs or cats, acupuncture on those points and a gold implant at one of the bladder specific points can aid controlling the incontinence in up to 90% of my cases. In few cases, like my technician's dog Linda, it can make the difference between being euthanized or being alive.

Linda was an orphan puppy that my technician rescued and hand raised. She was the cutest puppy, but had a severe case of urinary incontinence. This issue caused a lot of stress to the doggie housemates and her owner. We performed many diagnostics and suspected that her issue was a congenital situation.

Out of desperation to help her, I placed a gold implant, a 2mm small 24 K wire embedded under the skin at a special acupoint. It runs on the bladder meridian, on the lateral crease of the knee, called BL39. I also started her on an herbal formula specifically for incontinence called Suo Quo Wan. We were all pleasantly surprised when, within a week or two taking the herbs, she was 95% cured. I use gold wire implants as a last resort, but it has helped several pet patients control their bladder and live a normal life.

There are many factors in choosing the method to deliver stimulation to an acupoint. One of them is determining what kind of personality your pet has based on the Chinese Five Element Theory.

Take for example the **Wood,** or dominant personalities, are usually not very keen of being stuck with needles and staying quiet for twenty minutes. The **Fire**, which are friendly sweet personalities, until you put a needle on them. Then they scream or shake them off because they are extremely sensitive to needles and not great candidates for acupuncture. Lastly, the **Water** personality is the shy and fear biter kind of dog, which means that they will be very nervous and not enjoy the experience. The **Metal** and **Earth** personality types make the best patients for acupuncture!So what are the different ways in which Acupuncture can stimulate these very special acupoints in animals? There are several methods including Dry Needle (DN), Electroacupuncture (EA), Aquapuncture (AP), Moxibustion and Hemoacupuncture.

Dry needles (DN) refers to just a simple needle place into the acupoint. There are over 165 points to choose and the more points placed, the more diluted the effect of the treatment. In other words, a proficient acupuncturist rarely places more than twenty needles unless the patient has an Earth or Metal personality. There are many kinds and sizes of needles, which the acupuncturist chooses based on the intended therapy goal. Most patients keep the needles an average of twenty minutes, with the exception of kittens, puppies, and exotics. In those cases, the stimulation required is less than ten minutes because they are usually bundles of impatient energy.

Electroacupuncture (EA) Generally, for paralyzed or painful patients, I use EA because it is the strongest stimulation available. Basically, the acupuncture needles are placed and then, using some electric cables with clamps, attached it to an electrostimulation unit. This small device uses the power of a couple of batteries to send electrical energy into those needles.

Pet owners are often very surprised to see that those needles do not hurt their pets. I use peanut butter and treats to distract the pet while I am placing the needles. If a pet reacts to a needle, I am happy. Why? Because that point needed the stimulation and I just gave it. Pain is defined in TCVM as the blockage of energy (*Qi*). Therefore, the reaction when the needle is placed, known as *De-Qi*, tells the acupuncturist that her/his needle is in the right place.

Aquapuncture (AP) In chronic conditions or in very frail patients, I tend to use Aquapuncture, which is a milder stimulation. With AP, I inject a fluid bubble on top of the acupoint to stimulate it. The bubble gets absorbed within several minutes. My favorite solution to inject in AP is diluted vitamin B12, but many other substances can be used. Vitamin B12 has ample benefits for your pet, like appetite stimulation, increased energy, and improved nerve transmission. The vast majority of my cases start with twenty minutes of dry needles for the first six sessions, then are maintained with monthly quick AP sessions.

In some cases, I use a minute amount of other drugs. For example, I add Acepromazine or Valium when injecting in anxiety points for storm anxious dogs. I also try to use an appropriate acupoint when injecting antibiotics or any other injections in the skin. Other fellow acupuncturists also use blood drawn from the patient or just air drawn in the syringe in order to achieve the desired effect.

Moxibustion is the burning of a plant known to the Chinese as *Ai ye* and to the Western world as Artemesia vulgaris or Mugwort. This plant has healing properties because it aids in raising the energy of the affected area. Chinese healers use it to warm the Meridians by moving blood and *Qi*. I tend to place a little cone shaped piece of mugwort so it sits right on the acupoint with the needle in the middle. Sometimes, I just follow the Meridian along using a Moxa stick hovering above the skin.

More commonly, I teach the owners how to use Moxibustion at home due to the strong smoke it produces, which some of my staff is allergic to. We have a big laminated sign that says "MOXA in Progress". Several clients have compared the smell of mugwort to marijuana, which lends itself to funny assumptions. Moxibustion is sometimes used in conjunction with a human acupuncture technique called Cupping, in which the moxa smoke is used to heat glass cups that are then put on the skin to apply suction to the affected areas. This technique has gone mainstream after its success treating athletes during the Olympics. Unfortunately, due to the pet's fur and different skin architecture, cupping is not applicable for pets.

Hemoacupuncture- Finally, some points can be simulated by "opening" the channel using a needle to puncture it and allow some drops of blood to flow. This practice is called Hemoacupuncture and has some undeserved negative connotations, as it is sometimes confused with the practice of bloodletting.

Bloodletting is the process of bleeding patients in order to let the evil spirits out and was widely practiced from the times of the Roman empire until the early 1900's. Bloodletting was harmful to weak patients and not at all related to the proven benefits of Hemoacupuncture. It remains a valid treatment for certain conditions though, like Hemochromatosis, where the excess iron needs to be removed from the tissues and diverted into creating red blood cells.

The reason to use Hemoacupuncture is to clear heat from the Meridians. It's useful for cases of high fevers or inflammatory conditions, like certain autoimmunes diseases. The most common points I use are the tips of the ears and tail for cases with high fevers.

Another concept that people have some difficulty is with *Qi*. What is it? Remember we talked about energy in the last chapter? There is a vital force, an energy that exists in all living things. I know it sounds like I am talking about the "Force" from Star Wars ™ , and it is not a dissimilar concept. Cats and dogs don't duel with light sabers or move things with their minds. Or do they?

When a pet passes, their vital energy returns back into the universe. Here is what the famous physicist Neil Degrasse Tyson says on the matter. Remember the law of Thermodynamics, matter is neither created nor destroyed. That vital energy makes everything alive goes through the cosmic recycling program.

"The knowledge that the atoms that comprise life on earth - the atoms that make up the human body, are traceable to the crucibles that cooked light elements into heavy elements in their core under extreme temperatures and pressures. These stars- the high mass ones among them- went unstable in their later years- they collapsed and then exploded- scattering their enriched guts across the galaxy- guts made of carbon, nitrogen, oxygen, and all the fundamental ingredients of life itself. These ingredients become part of gas clouds that condense, collapse, form the next generation of solar systems- stars with orbiting planets. And those planets now have the ingredients for life itself. So that when I look up at the night sky, and I know that yes we are part of this universe, we are in this universe, but perhaps more important than both of those facts is that the universe is in us. When I reflect on that fact, I look up- many people feel small, because they're small and the universe is big. But I feel big because my atoms came from those stars."

— Neil deGrasse Tyson

Qi, the life force manifests in two mutually dependent forms, the *Yin* and the *Yang*. Modern physics and science agree that we are made out of energy. The Chinese knew this concept in ancient times and knew that the energy traveled in orderly pathways, called meridians. There are twelve main ones of those circulating energy around your pet's body. When the energy is blocked, thus not flowing, we consider that to be a disease process.

Pain is interpreted as the blockage of the *Qi* flow and acupuncture resolves this blockage by enabling the body to heal itself. Frankly, it is how we know when we have to go to the bathroom- we feel the urgency of a blocked flow. When *Qi* is blocked, we feel that pressure and pain.

Imagine a water balloon filled with water and you poke a hole in it, what happens? It explodes and you are all wet right? Ok bad example, as acupuncture does not make pets explode.

Imagine an irritation hose instead. It had all of these miniature holes that allow water to escape and reducing the water pressure inside the house. This is, in a simplistic way, how Acupuncture works, except it is Qi that you unblock.

IS ACUPUNCTURE SAFE?

It is a very safe medical procedure when administered by a qualified practitioner. In my experience, it takes an average of six treatments, one to two weeks apart for chronic conditions and twice weekly in acute cases, to have enough improvement that the owners can see that it's actually working. Each animal is different and, in Chinese medicine and acupuncture, that means the treatment has to be customized to the patient. As I've mentioned previously, there are no cookie-cutter treatments in acupuncture or holistic approaches. I do love to see the cases where we get truly dramatic results almost immediately because it makes believers out of skeptics.

PARALYSIS

Take for example the case of Bella, a Great Dane. She came in on a stretcher because she couldn't walk at all. I diagnosed a local pain and stagnation in the lower spine and treated her with electroacupuncture for thirty minutes. Amazingly, she stood up and walked out of the office! It definitively made her parents become avid fans of alternative medicine. Even my technicians were impressed. Some of the most common cases that I see are paralyzed animals. Several of them have been told that they need a quite expensive, in some cases $5000 or more, operation or they need to put their animal to sleep. I think that is irresponsible to say that to anyone. Even if you do not rely on acupuncture, medical treatment and strict rest could help the body heal. After some time resting and using anti-inflammatories and pain medication, many of them recover at least partial function. In worst case scenarios, a pet wheelchair is preferable to death, at least in my book. With acupuncture, you turn those odds around. We have seen up to a 95% rate of success in treating paralysis. I usually treat for a total of six weeks when I see a herniated disc.

Luckily, I've been blessed with several star patients experiencing incredible improvement from the first acupuncture treatment. Several have resumed walking after the first treatment. I recall a large Dachshund, my handsome patient Jackson, who came to me paralyzed. His mother was crying because she was scared that he would remain crippled forever. I put one needle on the tip of the tail and his tail wagged. Looking into her eyes confidently, I said he'll walk again. Imagine my surprise when three days later, she came for the second session with him standing by her side and starting to walk. His owner was very happy and this experience made her a believer in acupuncture.

In the few cases that acupuncture has not worked, I suspect an underlying condition like a spine tumor, a progressive disease like degenerative myelopathy, or a Fibrocartilaginous embolism in the spine. I have referred those patients to a neurologist who then confirmed my suspicions. Even with those incurable diseases, acupuncture can help by maintaining the muscle mass, help controlling pain, and promoting a sense of wellbeing.

KNEE INJURIES

One condition that I'm pretty skilled at and have excellent results is ACL knee injuries. I presented a scientific paper at the 2015 International Congress of TCVM on my method of treatment after high success rates. When I was in veterinary school decades ago, they taught me that ACL knee ligament injuries heal within three to six months by western medicine intervention and rest for dogs under thirty pounds. However, dogs over thirty pounds were often referred for surgery. In the paper I presented, I treated dogs of 18, 38 and 78 pounds successfully with aquapuncture using Vitamin B12, an herbal Tendon ligament produced by Jing Tang, and conventional painkillers or anti-inflammatories for the first week post injury. The owners were instructed to keep their pet quiet and to not allow their pet to jump. Amazingly, all of them regained full use or at least 90 percent use of the leg within three treatments.

A pleasant surprise at the 2015 World Congress of TCVM in Florida was that hundreds of veterinarians all across the World were seeing similar and even better results than mine using acupuncture for ACL injuries. Dr. Bruce Ferguson, a very esteemed acupuncturist, uses a minimal needle approach to all diseases and has helped hundreds of large and small animal with lameness and severe pain to feel better with just a needle or two.

Is Acupuncture successful as a 100% cure all of the time? No, but I feel that acupuncture can help 100% of the time, even if in differing degrees. For example, I have several cases of degenerative myelopathy, a disease in the spinal cord, where the spinal cord starts dying off and there is no cure. The standard prognosis is that the quality of life will be too poor and the animal is euthanized within three to six months post diagnosis. I still perform acupuncture and herbs on these patients because I feel that it helps to slow down the disease progress and keeps the muscle mass as long as possible. Basically, it gives the animal better quality-of-life longer and they are still living an average of one-year post diagnosis.

The owners can really see a big difference in their pet's general attitude and are very grateful for the extra time with their beloved companions.

HOSPICE CARE

Sometimes the cure is not what alternative medicine will give you, it's about quality-of-life and pain control. I always tell my clients what is important is not the amount of days that you live on this earth, but the quality of such days.

A large number of patients I treat are hospice care due to terminal cancer. These are very emotional cases, but end up being some of my dearest patients. As a matter fact, it seems that when you get a cancer diagnosis on your pet something amazing happens: people that would never consider acupuncture will open their minds enough to accept it. Maybe it is because they are desperately trying to save their pets or at least have more time with them.

Wilson, a beautiful Spaniel mix that was presented with a pot belly, difficulty breathing, and very weak, so much so he couldn't even walk. I took an x-ray of his chest and his lungs, which were filled with nodules everywhere. Although I did not do a lung biopsy, his blood work and the radiologist's opion was that it was metastatic lung disease from a primary liver tumor. The owner was devastated to know that he had such advanced cancer. I treated him with Stasis Breaker, which is an anti-cancer herbal formula, and acupuncture for hospice care. In cancer cases, the acupoints cannot be used near any tumor site because it will lend more energy to the tumor and encourage its growth. However, I use points that raise the immune system or increase energy in order to help the pets fight the cancer themselves.

Wilson kept getting better, being more active and happy, and his respiration improved greatly, I focused his acupoints to aid the lung and liver meridians and to raise his *Qi*. Three months later, I repeated the x-ray and could see his liver still was large, but there was a lot more normal lung tissue than before. His liver enzymes were better, but not yet normal. I told Wilson's mom that we would take it one day at a time and to enjoy him and allow him to enjoy life as well. Believe it or not, Wilson lived for four and a half years with pretty good quality-of-life.

Another example is my patient Dixie, who outlived the typical three to six months prognosis of Osteosarcoma and went on to live fourteen months of good quality of life. She was on regular acupuncture and Stasis Breaker as well! Her pain was controlled with an integrated approach using pharmaceuticals and acupuncture. Her points were mainly on the spleen and liver meridians. When I discussed this with my fellow teachers at Chi Institute, several of them told me that they had cases of Osteosarcoma live up to twenty-four months of good quality of life! I often tell my clients that as long as there is a spark and a will to live in their furry friend's eyes, we shall try everything available to help them!

Acupuncture can also help your pet make the decision to either fight and get better or to surrender and cross the bridge. How? There are special points associated with the will to live and the soul. I have used these points in cases where the owners are against euthanasia, but want to help the pet die with dignity and without distress. I put the soul points in and within twenty-four hours most of the pets pass away peacefully. Two have made incredible turnarounds.

I was caring for Leo, a sweet Sheltie puppy suffering from Parvovirus. This virus is a totally preventable disease when the puppies had their immunizations and come from mothers that had been immunized. Luckily, the pet owners realized that their brand-new puppy was sick and brought it to us in a nick of time. His white blood cell count was less than 1000 (the average is 5.5 to 17,000).

I hospitalized him in our isolation ward and used conventional medicines, antibiotics, immune stimulants, plasma transfusions, vitamin B & C injections, Aquapuncture and IV fluids. Despite all the medical care and TLC from our nurses, by the sixth day of hospitalization, the puppy took a turn for the worse. We called the owners and asked them to come visit their puppy to rally him up. I thought he needed a reminder that he had a loving pack waiting for him to get well. I also injected him with vitamin B12 on his "will to live" acupoint and started him on a high dose of an herbal medication called Blood Heat formula.

Imagine my delight when the next day, Leo was barking, wagging his tail, and moving around. Although he was still very frail, he made a dramatic improvement. Four days later, he finally got to go home.

Over the course of my twenty-two years of practicing, I've have to treat many parvovirus cases. I can tell you that a combination of acupuncture, herbal treatments, and positive involvement of the owners and my nurses have made the biggest difference in the outcomes and the speed of recovery. Needless to say, I use the will to live points in all my critical patients!

OTHER DISORDERS

Many people know that acupuncture helps with disc disease, lameness, and paralysis, but they do not know other conditions that can be helped by it. For example, gastrointestinal disorders like vomiting, constipation, and diarrhea can be helped with acupuncture. Cushing's disease, Hypothyroidism, Hyperthyroidism, and behavior problems are conditions where acupuncture is not commonly used, despite it being a great way to treat them.

Senior dogs and cats are like antique cars. When a part is broken, you fix it only to have another one break. That's the case with the hormones. They are in a feedback loop and if one depletes, it causes a domino effect. This explains how many senior diabetics with low thyroid and concurrent Cushing's are seen in my practice.

We can't keep substituting parts, and sometimes there are no replacements, so we must refurbish and maintain them. We are in a race against age and body deterioration and the best way to slow it down is using the holistic approach.

Quality-of-life maintenance and hospice care are often areas where acupuncture could provide help. Many of my cancer patients go on to live exceptionally long lives post diagnosis. Cancers have a common core of energy or *Qi* deficiency, and therefore the approach to "heal" is to replenish the *Qi*, especially the *Wei Qi*, which is the Defensive or Immune system *Qi*. If I cannot kill the cancer, at least I can erect giant walls of immunity to contain it and its damage.

As mentioned previously, the strength of acupuncture is in the prevention of disease, the management of chronic diseases, and the performance and endurance enhancement of animal athletes. Do not be afraid to reach for acupuncture and the holistic approach, they are just additional tools to help keep your pets healthy and live longer, better lives.

CHAPTER 6

HEALING WITH MASSAGE

• • • •

MASSAGE HAS LONG BEEN RECOGNIZED as a great way to relax muscles, release tension, and help you feel an overall sense of wellness. Pets experience much the same benefits that we do. In addition to feeling good, therapeutic massage can have positive physiological effects on the health status of the patient.

In western medicine, massage therapy has proven that it can improve circulation in affected areas, increase the massaged area's body temperature, relieve the muscle spasms and stimulate the sympathetic nervous system. It can also eliminate toxins by stimulating the lymphatics.

Through massage, we can also reset abnormally positioned anatomical structures, such as swollen muscles and ligaments. It is also used to effectively diagnose muscle tears and localize pain.

I am a certified *Tui-na* practitioner, which is a branch of TCVM known as manual therapy for prevention and treatment of disease. *Tui* means push and *na* means pull or lift. These techniques date back to the *Yin-shang* period, around 1600 B.C. In the world of TCVM, the whole body effects of massage involve the regulation of *Yin, Yang, Qi,* energy, and blood.

Through massage, you can unblock a Meridian and can also balance the internal organs. The local side effects of a massage in holistic and

TCVM is to invigorate the blood, remove the stagnation of blood and energy, eliminate swelling, relieve pain, and release spasms. Massage can separate adhesive tissue, which helps in the diminishing of scar tissue. The biggest benefit of this is the return to function of some joints and the improvement on the range of motion. Through massage, you could aid in vast different situations.

For instance, if you have an excess, which is a nodule or a swollen joint or a muscle that is having spasms or is out of place, then by pressing on it you can stimulate the sympathetic nervous system and help reduce the excess condition.

On the other hand, if you have a deficiency state, where your muscles are atrophying or the range of motion has been diminished, by manipulating, rolling, pressing, or rotating the tissues you can have a mild stimulus that may inhibit the sympathetic nervous system. At the same time, these actions stimulate the parasympathetic system which, increases the smooth muscle tone and circulation to those tissues.

Both western massage and Chinese *Tui-na* can be great therapies to help your pet with sore muscles, back pains, and arthritis. Veterinary chiropractic massage is similar to *Tui-na*; they have the same goal of treatment and prevention using manipulation by hands. Chiropractics focus on a local area and are pretty aggressive in manipulating the body, whereas *Tui-na* treats the whole body and is a milder manipulation. There are over two hundred technique styles of *Tui-na*.

What a lot of pet owners are not aware of is that massage can help with internal diseases as well. As an example, envision a situation where the pet has either diarrhea, constipation, or anorexia. Massage can improve the flow and rate of contraction of the intestines and relieve gas pain as well.

The TCVM theory explains the effect on the internal organs by the physical stimulation of the skin and muscle. The skin is dominated by the lung Meridian who's main function is to distribute the *Qi* through the body. Thus, if the *Qi* is flowing better through the body, the organs benefit because they receive the energy and nutrients needed to heal. There is a Chinese saying "*Qi* leads the blood". Wherever *Qi* flows, the nutrient rich blood is sure to follow. Another saying " where there is no free flow of *Qi*, there must be pain" adds insight as to how much we can relieve pain by manual manipulation of the skin and fur.

The other Meridian affected through manual massage and manipulation is the spleen. The spleen meridian is in charge of muscles and of generating the *Qi* from the food. A common sign your pet is not using a limb fully is that their muscle atrophies and gets thinner. By massaging the muscles and bringing energy and nutrition to them, we relieve pain and help those legs come back to function.

MASSAGE FOR PARALYSIS

Tui-na is an essential part of my recipe for any paralysis treatment. I teach the owner how to stimulate areas at home so that the effects of acupuncture are prolonged. There are very simple techniques that even less experienced pet owners can do at home to help their pet. They gain a sense of empowerment and participation in the wellbeing of their pet, which is priceless.

My patient Sadie, a long hair Daschund, was one of the first recipients of my *Tui Na* training. Sadie was totally paralyzed while I was on vacation so, she only received steroids and rest for almost a week until I came back and started her on acupuncture. She had lost all deep pain and had not improved on the steroid regimen. Along with electro acupuncture, I applied the few *Tui Na* techniques I had learned and saw immediate progress. It took eight weeks of hospitalization and daily massage, but Ms. Sadie walked again! She was featured in our local ABC affiliate news broadcast in a story on acupuncture being an alternative to putting paralyzed dogs to sleep.

CHRONIC CONSTIPATION

Many cats develop a condition called Megacolon, in which the colon loses the ability to move the stools out of the body and ends up packed full of feces. The colon gets very distended and the longer the feces stay there, the drier and harder they become. The colon wall may rupture or the toxins absorbed by the colon might make the cats very weak. In addition, the kitties are pained and refuse to eat. In some cases of severe constipation, the cats might try to eat, but vomit instead. Megacolon can be managed by feeding the cats only a high fiber canned food diet and administering motility drugs. *Tui-na* can be used along the ventral midline, the mid-underbelly, to help move the energy down and help move the guts. The touch needs to be firm and massaged in the direction of the flow, downwards. When we have these cases, we typically administer enemas and do a good belly massage, then hospitalize the cat until we make sure we have cleared the blockage.

JOINT CARE

One would think that massage is not good for acute trauma, but that is not necessarily the case. I've successfully managed many acute Anterior Cruciate Ligament (ACL) injuries with Aquapuncture and massage therapy. I remember one of my early successes was a seventy-five pound grumpy Pitbull with a painful ACL.

He hated acupuncture, but loved massage. We did cold water massage therapy with light touch for the initial sessions and after the swelling got better, the techniques became a bit more aggressive and decidedly warmer, which required firmer pressure and longer sessions.

With a combination of herbals and anti-inflammatories, he fully recovered and continues coming for regular massages for the past seven years. Now gray and slow, he still perks up when told he is coming to see us. Who can blame the guy for being excited at the prospect of having several pretty girls massage and love on him.

I have three certified canine massage therapists on staff for a reason, I truly believe massage is an integral part of a wellness and rehabilitation program.

PEDIATRIC ANIMALS

Pediatric animals are another great candidate for massage therapy. They are small and most pharmaceuticals are too harmful for them. Even using certain antibiotics could permanently affect their teeth and their joints. Therefore, baby animals can really benefit from the holistic and TCVM approach. I used *Tui-na* in a six-week old Pitbull puppy that was a rescued from dog fighting sting operation. This poor baby was paralyzed but was so small I could not use any of the western medicines.

She had a strong will to live. She would drag her little body to the food dish and growl at the other puppies to defend herself. I looked into her big eyes and saw a smart, determined look that warmed my heart. Decision made, I would do anything possible to see her get through. If I didn't, the despicable people that bred her and her family to fight would win. I used the smallest acupuncture needles (korean hand needles) and daily *Tui-na* on her spine and back legs. Imagine my joy when just within a week of treatment, we saw her trying to stand and walk!

We named her Gretel and continued to treat her until she walked again. Granted, she wasn't walking perfectly and her knees had reduced range of motion due to the tendons contracting, but she was a happy, hyper and playful pup. Her amazing survival story made the newspaper and inspired many people in my area to try TCVM. Do you know what the best part of her story was? Gretel found a great home and now lives the life of a diva. http://video.theledger.com/video/3918408116001#gsc.tab=0

Another pediatric patient was a four week old Maltese named Prince. He was paralyzed at birth, most likely a sequela of being breech, or stuck in the birth canal. The owner likely pulled to remove him from the birth canal, causing blood stagnation on his spine. I did acupuncture on him, but mainly showed the owner how to do *Tui-na* on his back and back legs. Prince recovered and walked again with just four treatments of acupuncture along with the herbs and daily *Tui-na*. The owners stopped coming for his treatment and a couple of months passed by. They eventually brought him back in and relinquished him to us. He was still walking and standing, but his tendons were contracted and limiting the movement of his knees. We immediately started him back on the TCVM regimen using electro-acupuncture and massage, and he started to regain most of the motion back. The owners realized that Prince would need a lot of continuing rehabilitation and surrendered him to my hospital. One of my technicians fell in love with him and adopted him. She still brings him to work with her and we provide holistic care. He walks, albeit crookedly, and is growing up to be a handsome and sweet little guy!

I mainly use *Tui-na* as homework for the owners. Whenever I am treating paralysis or any musculoskeletal condition, I try to involve the owner in the healing process. Generally, I give them one or two exercises to do daily. In my experience, you only need one to three minutes per exercise a day to see results. Take for example a cruciate ligament injury. In those cases, the ligaments that keep the knee joint functioning rupture due to a traumatic injury, most likely running and taking a wide turn. I usually do acupuncture, send the dog on the herbal formula Tendon Ligament (sold by Jing Tang Herbals, Inc.), and teach the owner to massage along the bladder meridian. This meridian travels parallel to the spine and supplies energy and stimulation to all the organs in the body, plus has several acupoints associated with pain control. The acupoint bladder 18 is around the tenth thoracic vertebrae, which is a very common area for disk problems, and related to the liver, which in turn controls the ligaments. When I demonstrate this technique to the owners, I ask them to go against the grain of the hair starting from the rump/buttocks and go up to the point of the shoulder for a total of ten times, five each side.

CONTRAINDICATIONS OF TUI-NA

The main contraindications of *Tui-na* and massage include fracture sites because obviously they are painful and you can actually move the alignment of the bones and worsen the situation. In very old animals, you have to be extremely careful with deep stimulation because their bones are very fragile. Pregnancy is another contraindication. Massage can be done, but preferably by an experienced massage therapist instead of at home caretaker. Some massage could stimulate the fetus and cause premature contractions. If there is a mass in the skin, it should not be massaged because it will promote circulation to the mass and help spread the cancer.

Any condition that causes dermatitis or infected, bleeding, ulcerated skin is another contraindication for massage. If it is infectious, do not massage as you could unwillingly spread it.

Another cardinal rule is to never massage after a meal! Ideally, you should do *Tui-na* three hours post meal, but if needed earlier, then at least wait thirty minutes!**Geriatric Conditions**

Tui-na is not just for joint issues and paralysis, there are many conditions that can be helped with massage. Sasha was one of my first successes with TCVM, she was an eleven-year old yellow Labrador that had lost almost twenty pounds from Inflammatory Bowel disease. She was very arthritic and weak in the hind limbs. She was vomiting up almost everything she ate. I treated her with acupuncture, homemade diet, herbals, and taught the owner how to massage the area in the mid-back (thoracic 10th vertebrae to lumbar 2nd vertebrae). She made a complete recovery and went on to live to the ripe age of sixteen! She had a monthly acupuncture appointment and received regular massage through all those five years. Needless to say, when her owner and I made the decision to let her go, it was a bittersweet moment. We agreed it was time and were grateful for the extra time and great quality of life she had.

Massage can be used in any arthritic or geriatric dog or cat under the direction and supervision of your veterinarian. It's a great add on modality to the treatment of chronic pain, chronic arthritis, and just for well-being. Massage can be used to shorten the time of healing and the diminishing of scar tissue formation by again softening the tissues and bringing in circulation to the affected areas. In essence, you are giving nutrition to those sick parts of the body.

It is a great bonding experience with your pet because they truly enjoy the attention and the relaxation that comes with a massage. In my opinion, walking with your dog and daily massages are two of the most important bonding rituals you could establish with your loving companion.

With every case of acupuncture, I usually teach the owner one or two *Tui-na* techniques to do at home. It is not a moneymaker for me, it is a tool for pet owners to continue to stimulate the meridians and acupoints that I jump started using acupuncture. Along with acupuncture, herbs and good nutrition, *Tui-na* completes the whole TCVM package for my patients.

10 EASY TUI-NA TECHNIQUES

Below are ten easy Tui-Na exercises. My pug Daisy was generous enough to allow me to illustrate them for you.

Yi -Zhi- chan= single thumb

This is a shaking technique that uses the tip of the thumb as if it was a needle and moves the rest of the hand as a pendulum. The movement is fast and applies variable pressure. I use this when I have a small area to treat that is very painful and deep. I remember using this technique on my own pet rabbit Clover that had a head tilt and painful neck. She acted like I was hurting her, but once I finished I saw an almost immediate improvement. Anytime you can pinpoint an area of discomfort like knees or hips, you can use this technique. Apply varying pressure;

firm and deep to shallow for about three minutes per area. Repeat twice daily until the pet acts less painful.

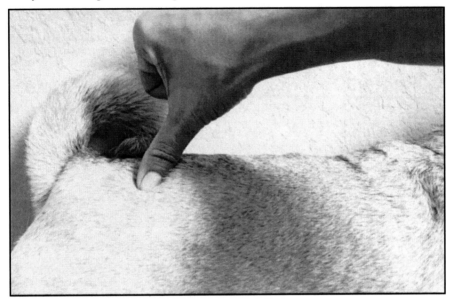

Rou-fa =rotary kneading

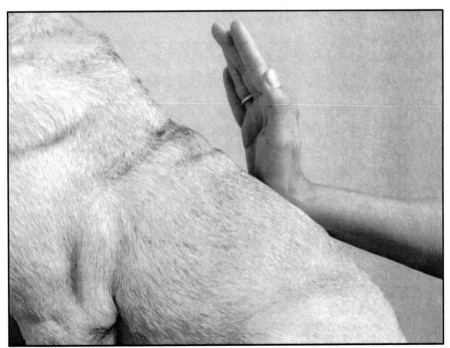

In this technique you use the palm of your hand and rotate on a point for about thirty seconds to a minute, moving alone until you cover the affected area. I teach owners of geriatric dogs to do this long each side of the spine (Bladder Meridian) and over the hip areas. Arthritis is the main reason to use it, but it can also be used on the belly to relieve stomach aches and indigestion. A daily session of three to five minutes is meant to be have a soothing effect and improve the circulation over those areas in need. Most dogs love to have this done.

Moo-fa= daubing or hello massaging

This one is called the "hello" technique because is usually the first one performed after meeting the dog. It is a face massage and is good to introduce the pet to your touch. I use it to gauge the pet's response and see if they grant me permission to massage them. It's the first step on any massage session and the pressure is medium, not too firm. It is done on the head around the eyes, temples, back of the ears and forehead for about three minutes. I use my thumbs with a gentle pressure going side to side or up and down in the same spot.

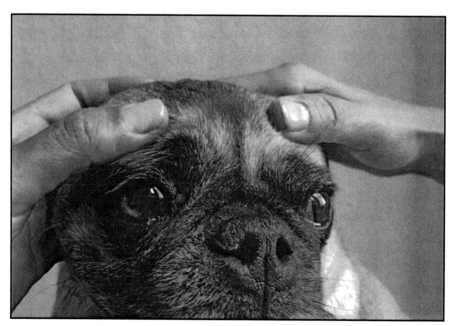

Ca-fa=rubbing

I use this for geriatric dogs that have a cold to touch area. The cold means there is not enough Qi (energy) in that area. Most times the rump and buttocks are cold on frail animals and a five minute session can warm them up. The way to achieve this is by using your palms with a fast and linear movement repeated over a static point until your palm is nice and warm from all the friction. I believe that in weak patients, you are actually transferring some of your good energy thus invigorating them.

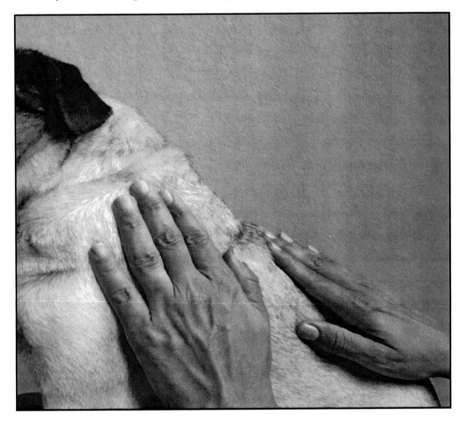

An-fa=pressing

This is a simple yet extremely effective technique. Using your fingers or the palm of your hand, exert moderate pressure on an area of good muscle mass, like the back. I advise to start light and continue to increase the pressure on the point. The pressure is meant to unblock the Qi thus is used for sore areas where your pet is reacting. Hold the position for one to two minutes.

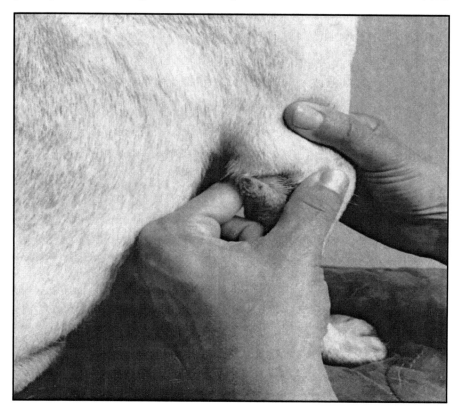

Nie-fa=pinching

This one brings up some child memories of my mom pinching my ears when I misbehaved, which rarely happened. It turns out that the act of pinching and squeezing then releasing the skin is a great Tui-na technique. This might be my number one prescribed technique that I recommend for at home care of sore arthritic backs. I usually tell clients to start at the base of the tail and move forward up to the neck repeating the movement daily for at least ten times.

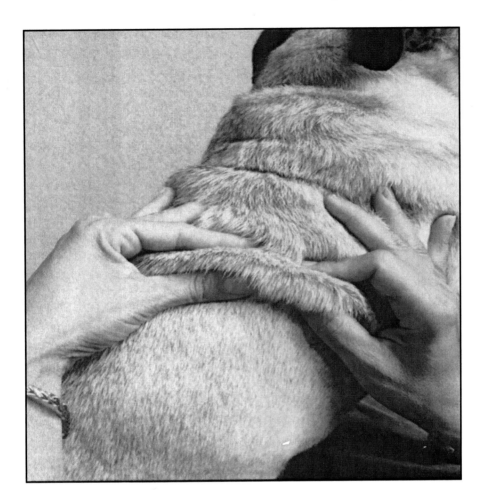

Dou-fa=shaking

If you've ever had a chiropractic treatment, you probably had this done. The technique is used for the weak limbs and the paralyzed ones. Basically, you hold up a limb with gentle traction then start rapidly trembling or mildly vibrating. It mimics a chiropractic move, but is gentler and can be repeated daily for three minutes per affected leg. The TCVM indications are to smooth joints and regulate Qi and blood.

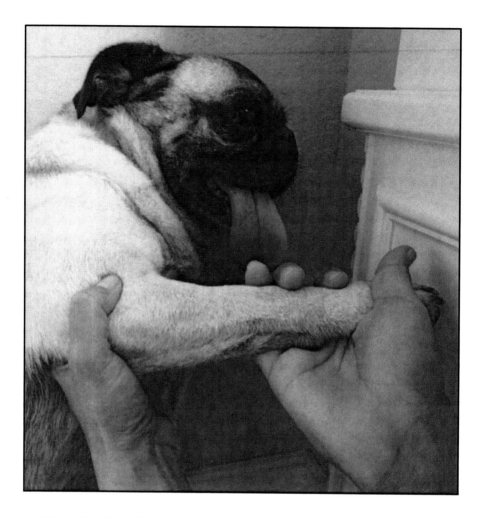

Zhen-fa=vibrating

This is a technique that uses higher vibration and can easily be achieved by using a home massage vibration tool. I recommend moving the massage head in circular motion along the affected areas. This one is a good one for chronically constipated dogs and cats and you can gently use the massage tool in their tummies. I also recommend this to be used on paralyzed dogs on the central or large pad of their back paws. An inexpensive rotary toothbrush can be used to provide this stimulation for just one minute per day.

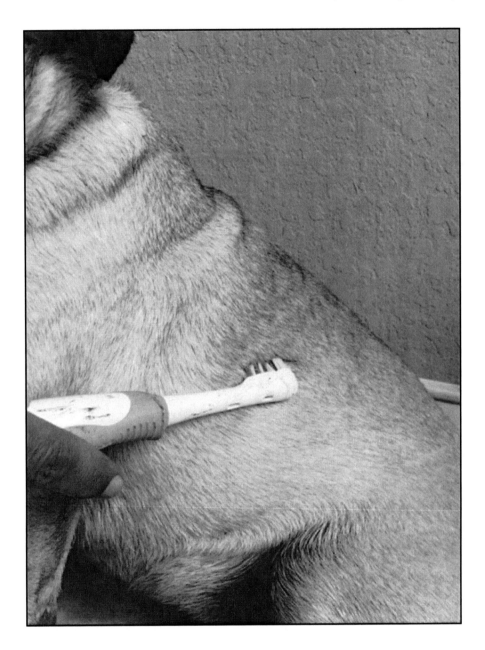

Pai-fa=patting

This is a great one for back pain and one of my favorites to have done on me. The nail salon I frequent has this in their chair massage and it is simply the best way to release back spasms. I teach owners how to do this one when I'm treating paralyzed animals. The fingers are together and the hand is held in a concave shape. The movement is fast and done as a rhythmic slapping of the tissues. The back, shoulders, rump, and major muscles are treated for three to five minute daily sessions. This one is noisy and should be done with soft pressure.

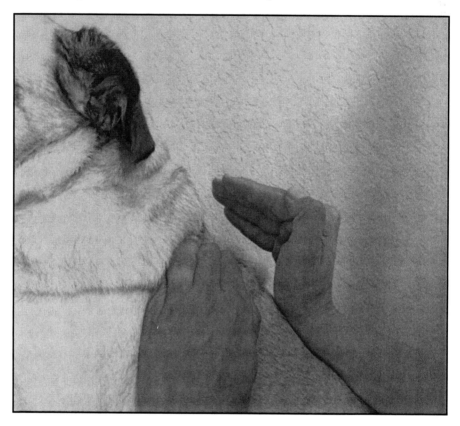

Ji-fa = beating

This technique is a standard feature of most human massages. The sides of both of hands are used in a rhythmic linear beating pattern along the back or hip areas. This exercise is great for arthritic pets and paralyzed ones. It looks like you are playing drums, just do one to three minutes per area daily in order to see results. The quick actions bring blood to the surface and have an invigorating effect.

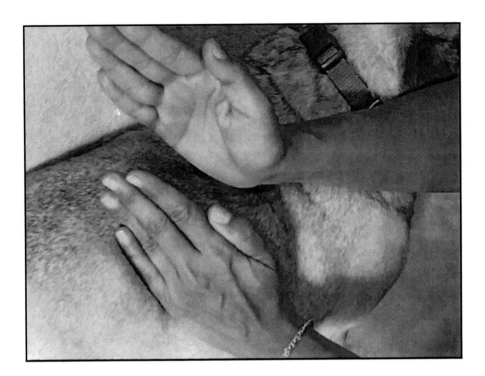

Massage therapy should be a relaxing experience for both you and your pet. Cats are also great subjects for massage as long as you respect their sensitive areas, like the base of tail and underbelly. In order to achieve your pet's cooperation, try to exercise them at least a half hour before the session. Do not feed them less than three hours prior. Choose a calm area of the house, minimize distractions, and place the pet on top of a comfortable blanket or rug.

You need to calm yourself and let go of your busy mind chatter. Touch with confidence and with deliberate intention to heal. Soft music or the sound of running water from a small home fountain can be great background noises. You can talk to your pet, but avoid baby talk or high pitched sounds as they tend to excite them.

Tui-na can be a great way to not only connect with your pets, but for you to be a part of their healing process.

CHAPTER 7

HEALING WITH FOOD

• • • •

WESTERN MEDICINE DIETARY recommendations are based on daily nutrient requirements which calculate how much carbohydrates, fats, proteins, vitamins, and minerals people and pets need. The TCVM Food Therapy concepts I am about to introduce you to are based on achieving health balance by eating foods with different flavors or energetic properties to help a pet based on their personality and the organ affected by disease.

It is important that you involve your regular veterinarian in the decision to use Food Therapy. Sometimes the recommendations for TCVM are in opposition to Western approaches. One of the biggest contentious areas is about Kidney Disease Management. My Western Medical training recommends that all cats showing kidney disease can benefit from being in a low protein diet. TCVM is looking at the energetics and does not take the protein content into the same consideration. According to TCVM, Kidney disease could have a root in many different patterns like a Kidney Yin or Qi deficiency and, in most cases, will find improvement using the adequate foods, regardless of protein content.

WHICH WAY IS CORRECT?

It depends! I have hundreds of kidney failure cases to illustrate this, but let me start with one from my pre-TCVM years. My sweet patient Taj was a Siamese cat that at age twelve, I diagnosed with kidney failure. I still remember how devastated and afraid her owner became when I showed her the blood work. I calmed her and told her if we could change her kitty's diet and support her with fluid therapy, we could achieve quality of life for a couple of years. She was treated using a mostly Western medicine, but the owner focused on diet, regular Vitamin B 12, and fluid therapy as well as nutritional supplements to help the kidneys along.

Taj would not eat the restricted protein diet and sometimes would have no apparent appetite, so I told the owner to continue giving her usual canned food diet, which was higher in meat protein. I told the owner to give her whatever canned diets she liked or chicken flavored baby food if she was being picky.

The reason I capitulated on the prescription diet was that is that it was worse for her not to eat than to eat a higher protein diet. She was very fragile and we needed to keep her stress free so I rejoiced knowing she was at least eating her commercial food and trying the supplements and fluid route. When I treated her, I had not yet learned about Chinese Food therapy, yet intuitively I knew that this kitty's body was craving something in that chicken can food that she needed. Envision my delight when she made it to twenty years old.

HOW DOES FOOD THERAPY ACTUALLY WORK?

Suppose that every single food item has a certain energetic property. You need to match the energetic imbalance that you are seeing in your pet with the food you are feeding them.

There are many ways to use the energetic value of food using TCVM concepts, but for the average pet owner I will limit my discussion to using flavor and temperature only.

FLAVOR

I can use the taste of the foods to match the problem with whichever one of the Five elements is affected. Foods could be Sour, Bitter, Sweet, Pungent, Salty or Bland. Each flavor can help solve specific problems. Let's look at how this can work for a common problem I see in pets, diarrhea. This problem can be caused by many TCVM patterns and it can be solved using totally different flavors of foods.

Sour dries up the body fluids. If your pet has diarrhea or urinary incontinence, then it makes sense to feed sour foods like tomato and pineapple. Vinegar and lemon juice could be added to the commercial food as well. Most pet owners feed boiled chicken and rice when they see that their pet has diarrhea. Why does it work? Chicken is a sour food, which will dry up the gut, and rice is a pungent food, which aids in relieving *Qi* blockages, which relate to pain. Therefore, boiled chicken and rice is the universal food balm for a sore GI tract!

Bitter takes the heat conditions and basically purges the intestines. In TCVM, heat is a pathogen and a disease causing agent. If your pet is suffering from diarrhea with bloody mucus, I assume there is heat present and would add some celery to the chicken and rice or may consider switching to ground turkey and rice instead.

Sweet foods are my favorite, perhaps because I am an Earth based personality, with a little Wood in it. These foods are the universal *Qi* tonics and providers of energy for all the internal organs. Suppose your pet is suffering from diarrhea and is very old. Because they are not digesting and eating properly, they will be prone to losing muscle mass and weakness. That is classic for a TCVM diagnosis of Spleen *Qi* deficiency, therefore, I would use sweet foods, like sweet potato, brown rice, or eggs, to help bring up the energy needed to tone the intestines so they can manage the job of absorbing nutrients and moving the bowels.

Pungent flavors activate the Qi and are very useful for pain and edema, swelling, conditions. Let's imagine your pet has a pain in their belly, and maybe he has flaccid guts with lots of air, or maybe the food is staying in the stomach too long causing pain. I would still use the chicken and rice, but I would also add a raw garlic clove to the food.

Salty foods soften hardness and also purge the intestines. So, I use salty foods when I have suspect tumors inside the guts that may be causing the diarrhea. I also use salty foods for the chronically constipated cats. Instead of chicken, I use crab meat, ground pork, or duck, keep the rice, and add some red kidney beans mashed into it.

TEMPERATURE

When it comes to using temperatures of the food to heal, the foods could be Hot, Warm, Cold, Cool or Neutral.

If your pet has an inflammatory condition, like allergic skin disease, you will see rashes and a skin that feels hot. I would recommend a diet based on a cold protein, like cod fish or duck. Tofu and Turkey are Cool, so they will also help. What I would never do is to put cat or dog on a chicken or venison, as they are Warm and Hot foods respectively.

Most of my paralyzed and arthritic senior dogs have back legs that feel cold to the touch. I see that as a need to increase their Qi/energy and add chicken or sweet potato to their diets and the changes I see are incredible!

What kinds of diseases have Hot patterns? Excessive heat in the body can sometimes be felt, as a part or the whole body will be warmer (swellings, ulcers, local inflammation) and/or seen (skin rashes, red skin, swollen red ears).

Interestingly, heat within the body can produce other symptoms unrelated to the temperature that we cannot see or feel. For example, a hot condition will dry up fluids which cause an array of issues. Let's say that if your pet doesn't have enough internal body fluids it can result in dried feces (constipation, megacolon), super concentrated yellow urine (Urinary tract infections, kidney insult), heat rising to head (swollen facial folds, dry mouth with sores, bright red tongues and gums, gingivitis, halitosis) and behavioral issues due to heat affecting the heart (storm phobias, doggie dementia, seizures, hypertension).

Where is this Heat coming from? It could be a result of eating highly energetic and dry diets with dry kibble or chicken. We are the sum of our environments so if your pet is living in a hot climate, it influences the internal temperature and puts a lot of stress on body systems to regulate the body. If your pet is under a strenuous exercise/athletic training, it will generate a higher body metabolic rate, which means higher energy and adds to the internal heat as well. Another way to increase the heat is due to a major organ malfunction, especially if the liver or heart are involved because the internal heat rising will cause seizures. Last but not least, senior pets undergoing "the hormonal change" will have a "false Heat" caused by a diminishing of *Yin* fluids like hormones, lymph, and blood. That pet will always be seeking to cool the body by laying on the tile, shade, laying around, panting, and drinking lots of water.

HOW DO WE TREAT HOT CONDITIONS?

Using raw foods or canned diets are the best choices because they contain much needed moisture. Cats are rare water drinkers, so a canned diet or at least a mix of can and dry kibble is best for them. In cases of inflammatory conditions in cats, tuna water or clam water may be added to their regular kibble or canned food. In addition, you can add electrolytes, like pedialyte, to both dogs' and cats' water to ensure they are properly hydrated.

TIP***I recommend putting unflavored pedialyte in an ice cube tray and freezing it, then add a couple of cubes to your dog›s water bowl.

Below are cooling food items that if incorporated in the diet can help heal hot conditions.

Fruits	Vegetable	Grains	Proteins
Apple, pear, banana, watermelon, cantaloupe	Spinach, celery, Eggplant, Kelp, radish, sweet corn, cucumbers, squash	Soy milk, tofu, mung beans, barley, Wheat flour alfalfa sprouts, brown rice	Turkey, Duck, Clam, Cod, Crab, Scallop, Rabbit

Let's talk about Cold/Cool Conditions affecting your pet. As I said before, the environment is influencing your pet's body at all times. If you live in a predominantly cold area, try to limit your pet's exposure to the outdoors or bundle them with a blanket so you help keep their inner warmth. The lack of exercise and resulting obesity is another reason to have Cold symptoms.

Your pet could also be born with a constitutional weakness, namely the breed traits, which will make it hard to compensate for the environment. For example, a Chihuahua was bred and developed for tropical and warm areas, thus you can imagine that living in Alaska would be putting an extra stress on his or her constitution. Eating too many cool/cold foods will result in a deficit of Heat (Yang) internally.

So, if you live in Alaska, feeding raw diets to our imaginary Chihuahua friend will predispose him to acquire a Cold pattern of disease. Excess Cold or Yang deficiency will manifest as affecting the Water Element in the Body, which in turn relates to the kidney system. The Kidney governs the bladder, kidneys, joints, the bones, and the sex organs functions. If we use water as an example, then we know that when water freezes, it contracts. If the body fluids cool down substantially, this may cause pain and stiffness in the joints. The pets will be seeking warmth by going under your covers, laying in the sun, acting hyperactive, or trembling.

HOW DO WE TREAT COLD CONDITIONS?

Simply using hot and warm foods that will help raise the internal temperature will help treat most Cold patterns. Dry kibble instead of raw foods is advised. Providing flannel bedding and keeping the pet indoors would be the best option.

Below is a table for Hot Foods that will help you warm up those cold disease patterns.

Fruits	Vegetables	Grains/Nuts	Proteins
Papaya, Peach, Apricot, Blackberry, Raspberry, Citrus, Plum, Coconut	Sweet potato, Pumpkin, Garlic, Horseradish, Ginger, Chives	Walnut, Nutmeg, Oats, White rice	Chicken, Venison, Lamb, Shrimp, Lobster, Beef Kidneys, Ham

HOW DO WE USE FOOD THERAPY FOR SPECIFIC DISEASES?

Liver disease is a common ailment due to the amounts of environmental toxins our pets are exposed to. It is also a consequence of chronic administration of medicines like Phenobarbital, Steroids, and Pain medications. I usually recommend to at least use one of my custom recipes to account for 20% of the total daily food given.

If the pet refuses my new food, I use single food items to achieve the energetic changes. If I have a TCVM diagnosis that means the liver is having a hot condition, then I would use spinach or mung beans or mushrooms as a single item added to the regular pet's diet.

LIVER DISEASES

Those items have a cool energetic nature, possess many cleansing anti-oxidants, and usually taste pretty good. My first case of liver failure was a Chocolate Labrador retriever named Dudley. He taught me so much! I have spoken about him in other chapters because his case was long spanning and the owners and I were very emotionally invested in him. We did a lot of research regarding supplements and tested the power of Milk Thistle, Vitamin B12, and the compound that helps heal the liver called S-Adenosylmethionine (SAMe) on him. SAM-e is converted by the liver into other substances that have powerful anti-inflammatory and *analgesic* properties.

I am so thankful to his owners for allowing me to treat him instead of euthanizing him on that fateful day. He came in with a bloated pot belly containing a liver tumor, had yellow eyes and skin, and was anorexic. The liver heat was manifested in the yellow color on his skin, eyes, and gums. Another sign of heat was that he was panting non-stop, his skin was dry, and his coat was very dull. He was also suffering of another pattern caused by the chronicity of the liver issue, the heat damaging his body fluids. If a pet has multiple patterns, I often clear any hot patterns first, as the Heat tends to consume the body quickly.

The recipe for Mung Bean Soup that I gave them was not only delicious, but it helped clear the liver heat and re-established his appetite. I was able to switch his diet to a *Qi* building diet while using acupuncture and the supplements to keep the liver going. The owners were impressed with the changes and decided to make homemade meals for their three other dogs. They were also glad that their dogs were acting more energetic and were generally healthier in appearance. It was very gratifying to know the profound change the owners undertook. They paid attention of what they themselves were eating and became a lot healthier as result. Heart disease is a progressive condition that could be caused by genetic predisposition, acquired diseases, or by simple aging. There are many good ways to diagnose and treat heart disease with western medicine. However, in the early stages of the disease or in the cases which have maximized the pharmaceuticals but are still having symptoms (coughing, weakness, and discomfort), TCVM using herbals and/or diet could bring a better quality of life. I would rather be proactive and tell all my clients how to do our best to avoid or at least slow down the progress of heart disease in their pet and a good, antioxidant rich diet is paramount to achieve it. When it comes to determining what kind of diet I recommend, it really depends on the TCVM pattern of disease I uncovered. If the issue is syncope, where the pet faints all the time, or lack of energy and stamina, I add warmer food items like venison and quinoa in addition to the fresh ginger. If the pet has a pattern of symptoms where they are irritable, pacing and have a weak heart, then I recommend foods that are cooling and will have some blood building characteristics. In these cases, I will avoid ginger because it would be too hot.

ISSUES OF THE HEART

The Heart is the Emperor in the TCVM system; as such it controls the blood and houses the Shen or spirit. When the heart is not working properly, it affects all of the other organs. I usually advise all owners to add heart friendly antioxidants, such as CoQ10 enzymes, Hawthorn Berry and Vitamin C, to their pet's diet. They can, in many cases, help reverse heart damage.

I remember my sweet friend Sport, the Bulldog. He lived a whole year past his terminal diagnosis from a board certified cardiologist. The owner was told there was nothing else they could do. By following some of the advice given here, we were able to extend his life and give him quality time with his beloved owner. There are many other patients that

I care for with early heart diseases that are being managed by an integrated approach (using herbals, acupuncture and food therapy) and showing that heart disease can be managed. Chronic cough can be a result of heart disease, asthma, bronchitis, lung worms, and lung cancer, among other conditions. There are foods that can benefit these coughing pets by lubricating the lungs (apple, egg whites, white sugar, ginseng), by stopping the cough (bitter apricot seed, kumquat, tangerine and thyme) or by toning the lungs (milk, licorice, sweet potato).

KIDNEY DISEASE

Kidney disease is another progressive condition that we have to deal with on a daily basis. Earlier in the chapter, I mentioned the protein dilemma regarding this disease. According to TCVM, among many functions, the kidney is in control of the bones, has the "source *Qi*" that makes all the other organs work, and is the reservoir of *Jing* or prenatal energy. Therefore, when an acupuncturist mentions the kidneys, they are not just talking about renal function or the state of the kidneys.

In reality, all my arthritic, paralyzed, and senior patients will suffer an imbalance in the Kidney Meridian. Regardless of the underlying pattern, a proper, custom diet along with fluid therapy can help halt the kidney damage and eliminate toxins. When it comes to kidney disease due to age, diet could prolong the life by adding quality, keeping the senior pet hydrated, and providing enough energy to compensate for the catabolic effect of kidney failure. Again, our sweet foods that are highly energetic examples will be beef, chicken, boiled eggs, and barley.

Even baby pets can have kidney issues. In fact, all congenital or hereditary conditions are thought to be a result of Kidney *Jing* deficiency.

If you are born with weak kidneys, then you are probably going to suffer genetic and congenital issues including weak teeth and deafness. The best way to improve this is by raising your *Qi* through high quality diets that tone, along with herbal formulas and acupuncture. The best news is that *Jing* disorders like Hip dysplasia, seizures, liver shunt, and infertility could all be helped, and in some cases be made clinically sound, using food therapy.

When senior pets get older, they show Kidney Yin deficiency, which is often characterized by incontinence, vision loss, weakness in the back legs, and insomnia. These could be addressed by feeding neutral or salty foods and in some cases mix in cool items. Examples are pork, beef, duck, millet, tofu, barley, and mung beans. I once had a small kitten that was brought to me because she had a condition similar to myasthenia gravis. Her esophagus was not working properly and she could not swallow her food. The owner was told to euthanize this kitten, but she came to me for a second opinion. I treated the kitten with aquapuncture and gave her a homemade recipe for *Jing* deficiency to be processed as a soft gruel and given as sole diet. Within six months of starting the food, the owner noticed she was much stronger and growing at an almost normal rate and she started giving a thicker consistency of foods. As one would expect this kitten recovered and is living a normal life.

ENVIRONMENTAL ALLERGIES

Allergies are synonymous with living in the eternal greenery of Florida. Our practice sees a large load of dermatological issues including allergies to fleas, food, and environment. The major Meridian affected is the Lung, which controls the skin. The itching is called external wind in TCVM and it is the single symptom that drives dogs and owners crazy. I have seen many a desperate owner that comes begging to stop the constant cycle of chewing-scratching.

Some allergic disease cases may follow the pollen loads and the seasons. It usually subsides from October to February, then comes back with a vengeance. A main culprit is fleas and, unfortunately, TCVM still doesn't provide new magic tricks to get rid of those pesky critters. Living in swampy Florida, where the fleas thrive the whole year round, we have tried using many natural remedies like garlic, neem oil, tea tree oil, moringa oil, oregano oil, thyme oil, brewer's yeast and citronella soaps with little success. Other causes of allergic disease or Atopy include environmental allergens causing Hay Fever. Instead of runny noses and postnasal drips like humans, pets get red or infected skins, itchy behavior, and ear infections.

Food can cause allergic disease as well. The main factors that contribute to food allergies are the kind of protein used and dyes or preservatives used in that diet.

Most red and itchy conditions benefit from cool/cold diets that have turkey, rabbit, fish, millet, or spinach in it. Foods that could cause allergic reactions may manifest in skin problems and ear problems as well. Other than consulting a pet dermatologist, doing an elimination food trial is something any owner could do. Just feed one specific diet exclusively; no treats, chewable meds, or table scraps for at least two weeks and if the skin starts to improve, you might be onto something. The majority of chronic skin infections and rashes could be alleviated using Cool Foods and switching the main protein of the diet.

One of the common culprits of the skin cases I see is chicken based diets. Chickens are grown pretty quickly these days, from hatchling to broiler in only forty-nine days. That means chicken is highly energetic and Hot. If your pet is living in a hot environment and being fed dry chicken kibble, it can be too much heat assaulting their body and it can cause ulcers, redness, moist lesions, and constant skin and ear infections.

I have many clients that came to in for a steroid injection to alleviate their pet's skin and left committed to feeding a different diet and trying supplements instead. The "superstar" skin supplement is Omega 3 & 6 oils found in supplements like organic ground flaxseed oil. They are natural anti-inflammatories and nourish the skin. If the pet has severe dry skin and pads, TCVM considers it to have a blood deficiency and supplementation with foods that are blood tonics like sardines, eggs, carrots, liver, and dates will be indicated.

ARTHRITIS

Arthritis is a result of the wear and tear of your pet's joints over time. However, a good diet geared towards nourishing the Kidney and Spleen systems will help control muscle atrophy and keep the overall strength up.Hot arthritic animals can benefit from raw diets in small amounts. Coconut milk and honey could be incorporated into some treats as well. Some TCVM patterns are caused by Kidney Qi deficiency, where foods are used to raise the energy and provide extra warmth. I usually palpate the back and legs of the senior pets using the top of my hands. If the skin is cooler there, it usually tells me there is a lack of Qi in that area. Why? Because energy produces heat and lack of heat means the energy is not flowing freely in that area.

In those cases, a simple change, like telling the owners to give dates and sweet potatoes as treats instead of milk bones or junky treats, could result in a much happier and active senior pet. Turmeric is one natural anti-inflammatory I advise owners to give. It is easy to just sprinkle over commercial diets or add to homemade diet recipes at cooking time. In addition, Omega 3&6 oils, kelp, and Vitamin C will help almost any senior with arthritic pain. Adding glucosamine, chondroitin, and SAM-e supplements can also improve the overall mobility and strength of these old pets.

DEMENTIA

Canine Cognitive Dysfunction (CCD), or doggie dementia, could be a condition that is very responsive to your pet's diet. Food therapy can slow down the progression and even prevent doggie dementia. Cooking for your senior or supplementing dog foods with Blood and Qi building foods will provide much needed extra energy. Cats can also get dementia, although it is more common for them to have in conjunction with hyperthyroidism and kidney failure. When cats show signs of senility, the first thing I recommend is a blood panel for a better idea of the situation. The same concept of feeding *Qi* rich foods apply to most of these kitties. Glucosamine is well known for helping increase joint fluids and helping arthritis, but few people know the value of adding kelp to both senior cats and dogs' diets.

Kelp is a great addition for older pets because it is loaded with vitamins and minerals, as well as iodine to help with thyroid function. It is a good natural source of vitamin E, which many believe is a key brain nutrient. To prevent CCD, I recommend starting these supplements at age seven for large breeds and age ten for small dog breeds and cats. If your elderly pet is exhibiting signs of early dementia, switch to a homemade diet and add vitamin E capsules at a therapeutic dose of 25 IU per pound. I also recommend adding huperzine A or Ginkgo biloba, which have been proven to improve focus and memory in people. The doses are empirical and usually off label, since they are human grade supplements. It is best to ask your veterinarian what dose and frequency they recommend since the strengths and formulas vary per product. There are many disreputable companies selling useless products so a veterinarian recommendation is preferable. It is also important to realize that not all human supplements are safe for pet consumption.

CANCER

Cancer is an awful disease that frustrates me to no end. In my twenty-two years of practice, I've seen the incidence of cancer among all pets rise. Some colleagues say diagnostics are simply improving, but I believe there is reason to be concerned. It used to be that cancer was mostly a disease of old senior pets or specific breeds, like Boxers and Golden retrievers. Now I find it across the board and have to always add it in my list of differentials.

Pets seems to be reflecting the trend in of cancer as people. The American Cancer Society website (www.**cancer**.org) claims that in 2016, there will be an estimated 1,685,210 new cancer cases diagnosed and 595,690 cancer deaths in the U.S. On the other hand, a statistic cited from a small animal oncology book *"Withrow and MacEwen's, Small Animal Clinical Oncology (5th edition) 2013"* reports that at least 4 million cats and 4 million dogs will develop cancer each year. Sadly, close to 50% of dogs over ten years will die of cancer.

I think the rise of cancer directly relates to the environmental toxins and the quality of the food. In TCVM, cancer is caused by a primary *Qi* deficiency. Our immune system in TCVM is called the Wei *Qi* system and, if weakened by stress, heat toxins, over-vaccinations, and food toxins, this *Qi* deficiency will result in the blood accumulating or becoming stagnant and forming tumors.

Food toxins are a touchy subject for the thousands of pet owners nationwide that lost pets or saw their cats and dogs suffer early kidney failure after the widely publicized pet food recall of 2007. The media coverage of this devastating event exposed the pet food industry's poor practices of buying substandard ingredients, that in some cases had melamine and cyanuric acid poisons, and using them in even the most expensive of pet food brands. I treated seven patients with acute kidney failure due to the melamine poisoning. Sadly, all died due to their limited kidney function. This pet food recall planted the seeds of distrust in the minds of pet owners and holistic veterinarians.

Food therapy can make a huge difference in the quality of life of pets afflicted with cancer. In some cases, I have seen animals live many years after a devastating diagnosis.

One of many examples was Reilly, a chubby, anxious, sweet, and hyperactive fluffball that began having fainting spells. I sent in bloodwork and did X- Rays and electrocardiograms, which showed he had some heart issues. My next step was to refer Reilly to my favorite cardiologist

Dr. Spier. He diagnosed Reilly with a heart based tumor and told the owner he could die unexpectedly at any time, a very poor prognosis.

The owners came back for palliative care and I put Reilly on a special diet, supplements, Shen Calmer herbal formula, and an anticancer herbal called Wei Qi booster. That was almost four years ago and he still comes for his daycare dates at the clinic.

BLEEDING DISORDERS

Bleeding disorders can also be helped with food therapy. If your pet has been diagnosed with a disease causing your pet to bleed, lose clotting ability, or consume its blood, as in autoimmune blood disease, hemangiosarcoma, liver failure, then supplementing with certain foods can help. By either providing rich nutrients that promote the production of new red blood cells or promoting coagulation, foods can make a major difference.

Great examples of coagulation promoters are:

» Kale

» Leeks

» Spinach

» Collard greens

» Parsley

» Celery

» Vinegar

» Persimmon

» Cuttlefish

Foods that help anemia include:

» Cooked liver

» Beef

- » Egg yolks
- » Oysters
- » Kelp
- » Green leafy veggies
- » Carrots

I have many patients living well after developing nearly fatal auto-immune hemolytic anemia and thrombocytopenia, where the body consumes their red blood cells and the platelets. They were treated with integrative medicine. I used foods along with allopathic treatments and herbal formulas to help these pets overcome these devastating conditions.

Food therapy is a great way to help heal disease in a holistic approach. This modality is the hardest one to be accepted in allopathic veterinary medicine because it does not follow their way of analyzing the food components. It might be a hard concept to swallow, but the energy of foods we eat are the energy that we become. "We are what we eat" is an important tenet of food therapy that has been proven right numerous times in the field.

CHAPTER 8

HEALING WITH HERBS

• • • •

When I was growing up in Puerto Rico, my grandmother "Mama" Juana Davila tried teaching me about healing herbs. She learned the properties of the herbs from her mother and claimed this knowledge descended from native Puerto Rican's called Tainos. She certainly looked like a Native American, with her long straight hair, aquiline nose, and a leathery tanned skin that made her seemed like an ancient guardian of mother Earth knowledge. She was barely 4 feet 10 inches tall and soft spoken, but her commanding aura was enough to stop any of us grandchildren in our tracks. I loved her deeply, with a child's innocence that elevated her to mystical deity; in my mind she knew everything.

She raised chickens and pigs and taught me a lot about farm animal care. She consoled me when I burst out crying after she expertly killed a chicken to make chicken soup for me. I had asked her for soup because I had a head cold and was feeling weak. I felt guilty that my request had ended the chicken's life.

As an adult, I've grown to distance myself from the philosophy that animals are solely for human use, but at that moment I truly understood how she viewed life. I still remember helping her harvest and roast coffee, letting it dry up in the sun on large slabs of stone. She had a healing garden and prepared teas and poultices upon request. My relatives and I would continuously visit share our issues including headaches, tummy aches, tooth aches and skin rashes. She would go pick the indicated healing leaves, stems, flowers, or seeds and provide her folk medicine remedies. How I wish I would have been able to record all her knowledge! I still remember going to her for a sore throat, watching her boil the mint leaves, use her special white cloth to filter the green tea, then adding honey and presto! I knew I would feel better pretty quickly.

I treasure the memories of my grandma guiding me to cut the new leaves of special herbs from her garden to make tea. She showed me which teas are good for sleep, Valerian and Chamomile, or to aid in cramps or muscle pains, she would give me tea made of a fruiting tree called Guanabana. I remember digging out ginger roots and turning them into ginger candy, which was good for tummy aches. Growing up in the seventies, I remember hearing of other folk medicine "curanderas" nearby. They knew a lot more than my grandma and often charged for their remedies. These experiences ingrained a deep respect for natural cures and imbued me with love for mother Earth. I am very glad I found a path to finally start studying herbs and their beneficial effects.

Chinese Herbology might have started as folk medicine, but the anecdotal experience was passed down since and written since over 2,000 years ago. Modern science is taking a new look at these folk remedies trying to find and extract the active compounds that make them medicinal. Unfortunately, the method of preparing these herbs will definitely affect their properties, which means it is hard to reduce all their power into just a pill.

HERB THEORY IN TCVM

Herbs have different properties and a veterinary herbalist will use them according. There are many ways to use herbs, but I use the TCVM Five element theory, which recognizes five different categories of energy called Wood, Fire, Earth, Metal and Water. There are special herb properties that can be used to treat disease in any of those elements. Among those properties, I use temperature (hot, warm, neutral, cool, and cold), taste (salty, bitter, pungent, sweet, sour) and the twelve meridians they affect.

HOT AND COLD HERBS

The theory of herbs is similar to the one for food. When I use temperature of the herbs, I am basically trying to reach a balance by using the opposite temperature. If a condition is cold, then I try a hot herb and vice versa. If I see a pet with a high fever, I will use special acupuncture points to reduce the fever and prescribe a cold herbal formula to help as well. Simple, right?Say for example I am treating a case of acute bloody diarrhea. That is a hot condition that needs an herbal formula containing cold herbs like Coptis (*Huang Lian*). This formula is given until the diarrhea resolves. If continued after resolution, it could cause a cold condition to manifest. A cold condition in the intestines could also be diarrhea, but it has a quite different presentation. A "cold" diarrhea would be usually worse in the morning, might be chronic, and would be very watery, without blood or mucus in it. In that case treating it with Coptis would be a disaster! Instead treating with an herbal formula containing a Hot herb, like Cinnamon bark (*Rou Gui*), will help clear the issue.

	Hot Herbs	**Cold Herbs**
Conditions	Cold body parts, watery stools, Urinary incontinence, Nausea, Vomiting	Fever, Dry mouth, Infection, Inflammation, Sweating disorders
Examples	Aconite *Fu Zu*, Cinnamon *Rou Gui*	Coptis *Huang Lian*, Gypsum *Shi Gao*

THE FIVE FLAVORS

When it comes to using taste, each of the five flavors have specific effects that can be applied to treat conditions.

Flavor	Properties	Examples	Uses
Bitter	Clear heat based conditions and purge the intestines	Coptis *Huang Lian* and Rhubarb *Da Huang*	I use Coptis for acute bloody diarrhea cases and it is extremely effective and detoxifies the intestines within 48 hours. The chemical ingredient responsible for the good effects of Coptis has been isolated as Berberine and turned into a pharmaceutical. I rather use the plant source.
Sweet	Organ Failure	Ginseng, Licorice, Astragalus,	Tonifying Tonic, older, weak animals
Salty	Nodules and tumors	Minerals containing salts	Treat Cancer in Pets
Pungent	Stimulates the blood flow and wherever the blood flows the *Qi* will surely follow.	Cinnamon	I've read many articles on weight loss that praise the ability of Cinnamon to raise metabolism and aid in burning fat.
Sour	They are astringent, which means they stabilize and bind the substances (blood, sweat, mucus).	Schisandra *Wu Wei Zi*	Stop diarrhea, excessive sweating, and fecal or urinary incontinence

USE THE RIGHT REMEDY

Knowledge of the meridian affected is essential for finding the correct herbal formula. Therefore, a doctor well familiarized with TCVM is of utmost importance. You can't just choose a Chinese herbal formula based only on a western diagnosis. That is a recipe for disaster! In the first chapter, I explained how two pets with the same urinary incontinence diagnosis were caused by two totally different TCVM patterns. Special care must be taken when integrating pharmaceuticals with herbal formulas as well.

Take for example heart disease. If the pet is already on cardiac medications I usually find the TCVM pattern. After carefully evaluating the formulas, I start using a smaller dose of medication. Such is the case of my dear buddy Sport the bulldog- RIP. He was one of my all-time favorite patients and was a rescued purebred that had lost an eye. His pet parents were fabulous and Sport lived a wonderful life until he developed heart failure at the age of nine years. I sent him to a great cardiologist, Dr. Spier who said he was in advanced stage of heart failure. Though he put Sport on medications, Dr. Spier gave the pet owners a poor prognosis and recommended euthanasia. The owners knew how much I loved Sport so they called and decided to drive to our hospital for me to put him to sleep. When I saw him, I couldn't bring myself to do it. He put his face on my leg and I saw a spark in his eye; he was a fighter. I performed acupuncture and put him on Heart Qi tonic instead. We kept the regimen prescribed by Dr. Spier. A year later we celebrated the accomplishment of his tenth birthday. He lived several months past it until he earned his wings.

My grandmother and ancient Chinese herbalists knew certain herbal combinations were not good for the body. A competent herbalist knows there are rules about mixing herbs that need to be followed. I do not advocate the use of internet sources or just mixing herbs and supplements without consulting a holistic veterinarian. I once had a client whose dog was arthritic, panting, drinking a lot of water, and barely sleeping at night. I diagnosed him with Kidney *Yin* Deficiency, which means the cooling ability of the body was not working. I prescribed a formula, but the dog was not progressing as well as expected. When I asked the owner if she had started any other supplements, she answered that she did add garlic, for flea control, and ginger, because she heard it was good for stomach issues. Well, in her dog, those two food items were adding heat to an already hot body. It was counteracting the herbal benefits. We stopped the supplements and the panting and night insomnia resolved.

In general, herbal formulas are balanced and depend on the healing actions of multiple herbs. Often this makes them a little safer and more powerful than treating with a single herb. When you combine herbs, you can achieve a myriad of results. You discover herbs that assist the therapeutic effects of the principal herbs or you can add herbs to counteract the toxicity of the main herbs.

COMPLEMENTARY MEDICINE APPROACH

In most cases Chinese Medicine Herbs can be used along with western prescriptions without any ill effects. The biggest exception is cardiac and hypertensive drugs, since adding Chinese herbs with similar effects could create adverse reactions.

TREATING SEIZURES

When I see a patient that had a seizure episode, I first assess the need for prescription anti-seizure drugs. If the seizure was mild, the pet did not lose consciousness and recovered quickly, I do not reach for phenobarbital right away. Instead, I run blood work to rule out underlying causes of the seizures, like a low thyroid or bad liver. Then I perform a thorough physical and neurological exam and start them on an herbal medication and aquapuncture for seizure control.

If the episodes were severe or came in clusters, I will use conventional drugs to stop the episodes, but use TCVM along them. The ultimate goal in this combination is to eventually wean off the drugs or at least use minimal dosages. Therefore, it is very useful for owners to keep a log on the seizure activity frequency, duration and characteristics, like involuntary urination/defecation/consciousness, and share it with your veterinarian.

I've had many successful management of cases in cats, dogs, and even a gerbil using herbals. The main benefit is that not only are we controlling the symptoms, but we avoid side effects, making herbals a safe, lifelong treatment. I use five local points on the head to calm seizures and teach owners how to try acupressure on their pets. The holistic approach also involves changing the diet and adding some "brain vitamins" and antioxidants to ensure optimal brain function.I tend to prescribe herbs to tonify all the deficiencies created by the long term use of western drugs. That is my approach to seizuring dogs and cats using phenobarbital with or without other anti-seizure drugs who are still having seizures. I never take them off the phenobarbital right away; I usually add the anti-seizure herbal formula called Di Tang Tang and work on finding the root cause of the imbalance causing the seizures. I might also add herbs to aid and protect the liver from phenobarbital toxicity. Ultimately, my goal is to slowly wean off or minimize the dosage of pharmaceuticals and use herbs to handle the issue long term. I have a large amount of successfully managed seizure cases. I treated a Persian cat that was having seizures daily. When they gave the first pill of Shen Calmer herbal formula, the cat stopped immediately and regained a better quality of life.

My sweet patient Willie is another good example. I started him on Di Tan Tang, which controls seizures by removing phlegm from the brain. The seizures began to diminish in intensity and frequency, but it took a few tries to adjust the right dose of herbals. The good thing was even though it took the high end of the herbal dosage, all the seizures stopped and Willie's quality of life soared. I was confident that a high dose of herbs would still be safer than a low dose of phenobarbital. He has only proven my theory correct. Seizures are unnerving to pet owners and there are a myriad of underlying causes at the root of the issue.

Another patient was Kurley, a two year old Boston Terrier who was having continuous, hourly seizures for four days in a row when the owners consulted me. He was on high doses of Phenobarbital, Valium, and potassium bromide, but he could barely walk and was extremely weak. I took him off Valium, cut the potassium bromide dose in half, and started Di Tan Tang along with Wei Qi booster. As he progressed, I kept adjusting the dosages and eventually eliminated potassium bromide altogether. His daily seizures clusters stopped and although he still gets occasional seizures, they are much milder and hopefully in time they will disappear altogether. He is currently down to a half dose of phenobarbital along with the herbs.

The ideal patient should have a complete neurological work up with a specialist, including an MRI. TCVM can be used as an adjuvant or as sole therapy for seizure disorders, but an attempt to find the root of the issue should always be tried. One of those thoroughly worked up cases was Fonzi, an Italian Spinone gentle giant. He was on super high doses of five different pharmaceuticals and still having seizures. The owners had an MRI done and a focal encephalitis was diagnosed. The owner was interested in trying alternative medicine. I set a goal to first control the seizures with the herbal formula Di Tan Tang and then wean him off the other pharmaceuticals within a year. We are halfway through the year and had wonderful progress eliminating two pharmaceuticals and achieving great seizure control. We noticed that his seizures coincided with full moons and have since increased the herbal the day before or after any full moons. I suspect that since the full moon is the highest *Yin* energy time and his seizures are rooted on a *Yin* deficiency so his seizure threshold is the weakest at those times. So far, my theory seems to be working in stopping seizure activity.

HERBS ARE NOT ALWAYS THE ANSWER

Most pharmaceuticals such as antibiotics and anti-inflammatories appear to take effect much faster than herbs do. In acute situations, I will often reach for the quick effect of western drugs. When it comes to dosing the herbs, most of the information is empirical because there are many factors affecting the right dose. For the holistic and TCVM approach, you must take in account the right TCVM pattern causing the symptoms, the GI sensitivity, whether there are other underlying issues present, and any medication being taken concurrently. If my patients react to the herbs, I often tell the owners to halve the dose and see if that works. If it doesn't, I stop the herbs and wait three days and then give another half dose. If they have vomit or diarrhea, then I switch the formula. I've learned to listen to their bodies and take the way they react to further refine my diagnosis.

In my experience, purebreds are more sensitive to herbal therapy than mixed breed pets. Geriatric pets are also at risk of being overwhelmed by the herbs so I tend to start at 1/4 the optimal dose and build up until reaching my desired dosage. The standard duration of treatment is one to three months, but I often switch formulas and keep some patients in herbals long term.

CANCER

In cancer patients, I often keep them on anticancer herbs for the rest of their lives to prevent recurrence.

One such case was Mandy, the amazing Bichon Frise. Ms. Mandy lived a great life six years after being diagnosed with an inoperable nerve sheath tumor. I met Mandy's mom because she was told to euthanize her beloved baby and couldn't do it. The fact was that Mandy was an alpha, happy go lucky girl and was not ready to go. Unfortunately, she did not like having acupuncture either. I told her mom I could debulk the tumor to allow use of her leg and we needed to keep her on the herbal formula stasis breaker. In addition, I prescribed coQ10 enzyme and turkey tail mushrooms. She kept the tumor at bay and enjoyed her life until her last day on Earth, six years later.

I will never forget Abby, another kind Labrador, that fought oral melanoma and lived a blessed life two years post diagnosis. Her mom cooked a bone marrow recipe and fed it daily along with the anticancer herb Stasis Breaker. That case showed me that the best approach against cancer is to rally the patient's immune system against it. I also used an herbal formula called Wei Qi Booster and recommended a home cooked diet with antioxidant supplementation to do that. She ate, played, and enjoyed a great quality of life until the melanoma invaded her jaw bone. When compared to previous cases I had treated using allopathic medicine, Abby outlived them by one and a half years.

The way I apply TCVM to treat cancer varies from case to case. Sometimes we achieve reduction of the tumor size, or slow down the progression, and a few times, remission of the cancer. I can say that in most cases the energy is returned and the pets appear and act happier. Most cancers have a common core of energy or *Qi* deficiency, therefore the approach to "heal" is to replenish the *Qi*, especially the *Wei Qi*, which is the Defensive or Immune system *Qi*. If I cannot kill the cancer, at least I can erect giant walls of immunity to contain it and its damage.

For example, in my kitty patient Kiyah, a cat with stage four mammary carcinoma in both mammary chains, I did not pursue surgical options because the cancer was so widespread.

I simply recommended the herbal medication Stasis Breaker and pain control. She lived over two years of great quality of life, even when the pathology report suggested a poor prognosis of six weeks survival. The lung metastasis was delayed and the invasion of cancer into other systems was so slow that it allowed her a nearly perfect life for over twenty-four months. Her owners were grateful that the very inexpensive and non-invasive treatment allowed them to enjoy her company for two more years.

In these cases, the cancer was not cured, but that is not my goal anyway. My goal is to help my patient's immune system into containing the cancerous cells, extending their enjoyment of life, and their time with their pet parents.

POWER OF HERBS

I am humbled every day by the power in plants. Take the example of my dear client Margaret and her wonderful King Charles Cavalier, Ariel, who suffered from one of the worst cases of hip and elbow dysplasia I had ever seen. If you were to see Ariel run into our practice to get her monthly acupuncture you would think I am exaggerating. Fortunately, Margaret has been a big believer of the holistic approach, since she is originally from India and very knowledgeable in Ayurvedic medicine.

Over the past five years, she has allowed me to treat her beloved dog with stem cells, acupuncture, cold laser, gold implants, herbal therapy, massage, and food therapy. One root powder Ariel consumes with all her meals is the amazing spice known as Turmeric. I credit Turmeric, along the herbal formula Body Sore, a blend of herbs that act like a benign aspirin, with keeping her joints from swelling and getting stiff in between acupuncture sessions. She has had up to six month periods without needing to be seen for any lameness or pain, and is living a full and joyful life. She gets to eat a homemade diet along high quality grain free canned food as well.

The reality is that Ariel was born with severe hip and elbow dysplasia. Her hip sockets never developed, leaving the head of her femurs "floating" and creating a weak back end. Her elbows also are mildly deformed so she can't get relief by shifting all her weight to the front. This condition is usually treated with surgeries to amputate the head of the femur or surgery implantation of a hip replacement.

In her case, we have avoided any surgical intervention and kept her comfortable and out of pain using an array of alternative procedures and medicines. It is amazing to look at the horrible hips on her x-rays and see this sweet hyper dog wagging her tail at you.

I have so many patients that routinely use herbal formulas to aid in control of a myriad of diseases, from seizures to kidney disease. I add raw herbs like Turmeric, seaweed, or ginseng for severe arthritis in older patients. The approach to pain has to be multi modal. In other words, no one single treatment can safely eliminate all pain thus, we should use a combined approach by using traditional western medications along with dietary supplements, herbals, acupuncture, laser, and *Tui-na*.

One of my favorite herbs is milk thistle, a common herb used worldwide to detoxify the liver. The flowers of this plant were made in poultices and given to treat mushroom intoxication as early as two millennia ago. The plant thrives in the Mediterranean and Middle East and is featured in many folk medicine recipes in European countries. Modern pharmaceuticals have been made from the extract of these plants and the active ingredient silybin has been touted as an effective liver rejuvenator. I use it extensively, both as the pharmaceutical preparation and as the flower extract sold in my local health food store. In cases of severe liver failure or cancer, I immediately add milk thistle with or without the Chinese Formula Liver Happy.

SOURCING HERBS

Are all herbal formulas created equal? Not even close. The United States Food and Drug Administration (FDA) oversees the supplement market and Chinese herbal formulas fall under their umbrella. I only buy from Jing Tang herbals and Khan Herbs. Both these companies manufacture here in the U.S.A. and are considered current Good Practice Manufacturers (cGMP) that adhere and exceed the FDA standards. I caution owners against using Dr. Google for diagnosing pets or using unknown products bought from obscure Internet sources.

Some herbal formulas may contain ingredients like Aconite and Ma

Huang (Ephedra) and could be extremely poisonous or even fatal to your pet!

ADMINISTERING HERBS

How you actually give the herbs is a whole other topic. Any medicine is ineffective if the pet won't take it, right? The formulas come in liquid decoctions, loose powder, tea pills, and capsules. Every pet is different, so you might need to try a different type before you find the right one. When it comes to administering herbals, use peanut butter or hide it in a favorite snack. As long as there are no allergy concerns, the good healing power of the herbs trumps the extra calories of the sneaky delivery. In some cases, where coma or vomiting make oral administration impossible, I've even administered herbs rectally.

Herbal therapy can help manage a vast array of diseases. It can also prevent disease and help your pet live healthier and longer. Remember to ask your veterinary herbalist about side effects and contraindications of the herbs prescribed. Disclose ALL medications and supplements along with the diet that your pet is taking. Keep your veterinarian informed of all physical, behavior, or routine changes in your pets since starting on the herbs. Keeping a simple journal can help in figuring out the best dosage for your pet. Remember that disease patterns change and adjustments on the herbals dose and frequency might be needed.

Ten Medicinal Herbs that can help heal your pet:

1- Chrysanthemum *Ju Hua*

This plant is an ornamental, but the dried flowers are considered a superior herb. Chrysanthemumhas numerous benefits for the Lung and Liver channels. While it can be used as a single herb due to it being non-toxic, but it works better in combinations. It has been used in many sore throat preparations for humans, especially when combined with menthol. Chrysanthemum works great for liver Fire, or inflammation, since it is a cool and bitter herb. This herb is used in many traditional

Chinese formulas that can be used in dogs, cats, and horses. It can be prepared as a tea and given with honey for animals that have acute cold signs showing red eyes, sore throat (abnormally hoarse bark/meow), and dry non-productive coughing. This is a very popular tea used in China to prevent infections. Interestingly, studies have proven that the extract of this flower can kill the common bacteria Staphylococcus and the fungal organisms that cause ringworm infection.

2-Scutellaria or Skullcap *Huang Qin*

If you have a damp condition, which involves anything oozing excessive fluids, this plant will help drain it. It clears toxins and heat from the body and has been used to stop bleeding. Some use it to calm the fetus and stop miscarriages. The energetic properties are cold and bitter. The part used is the powdered root and it affects Liver, Lung, Gallbladder, Stomach and Large Intestine Meridians.

3-Rhubarb root *Da Huang*

This is a purgative herb used to expel toxins from the Spleen, Stomach, Large Intestine, Liver, and Heart. If a pet has jaundice, this herb will help calm the gallbladder and eliminate the bilirubin. Due in part for its ability to move the blood and remove stagnation, it is not recommended in pregnancy. I like this herb for constipated patients, but avoid using it as a single herb.

4-Ginseng *Ren Shen*

This is a beloved root by the Chinese that has been used for thousands of years. The energetic properties are warm and sweet, which are great for patients in shock. Ginseng replenishes the Qi and also calms the mind. It is a very strong herb and can have side effects if used as the only herb. The major effect is in the Heart, Spleen, and Lung meridians.

Weak animals and the geriatric patients will benefit from supplementation by showing increases in their activity level and getting better quality of life.

5-Licorice root *Gan Cao*

This sweet root is widely used in most herbals recipes as a harmonizer. When used as a single herb it can have serious side effects, but used in small amounts as part of a balanced formula is extremely beneficial to all the twelve Meridians. This herb clears heat and can actually help clear food poisoning. I advise it for animals suffering from chronic diarrhea, poor appetite, and fatigue

6-Seaweed *Hai-Cai*

This herbal is being harvested for use in a wide array of nutritional supplements. The powerful antioxidants can help with cognition and inflammatory conditions like arthritis. This bitter and salty energy herb is used in Chinese medicine to transform phlegm, which means it can help when used to reduce masses. I recommend seaweed for any prostate issues and for management of swelling and inflammation caused by chronic arthritis.

7-Ginger *Sheng-jiang*

Have you ever wondered why raw ginger is served with sushi? It is because ginger is a warm herb that is anti-vomiting and also help clear toxins. Since sushi is a cold food, it can cause stomach *Qi* to stagnate. Ginger balances the energies and prevents a tummy ache. I have successfully used a pinch of powdered ginger on top of dog food to treat chronic vomiting in dogs. However, you must make sure your dog is not having a hot condition as Ginger will make it worse. Any arthritis pain caused by cold conditions will benefit by using ginger.

8-Mint *Bo He*

Mint leaves and stems are very popular in teas and topical throat medicines because of its cooling effect. Mint is great to clear fevers because it promotes sweating. I've used essential oils when trying to prevent colds and some clients have used a small amount in their pets with good success. The strong aroma might be a problem for kitties, so I prefer to used it diluted in Chinese herbal formulas and not as a single herb. The main Meridians affected are Liver and Lung.

9-Cinnamon *Rou Gui*

The bark and twigs are used in Chinese herbal formulas. Its main action is to warm the interior of the body as well as the Kidney, Spleen, Heart, and Liver Meridians. The bark promotes great circulation and stops pain caused by cold conditions. In Western Medicine, cinnamon is used to increase metabolism and aid in weight control. Use carefully if your pet has a hot condition.

10-Turmeric

This is a popular herb that commonly used in Indian food and curry. The roots are dried and processed into an orange colored powder. I use it in my own cooking and prescribe it for arthritic and geriatric patients. There is a lot of evidence that the active ingredient in Turmeric, curcumin, is a potent anti-inflammatory and antioxidant. I tell my clients to sprinkle or add it to their homemade diets.

CHAPTER 9

EMERGENCY RESPONSE

• • • •

Disclaimer: The contents of this chapter are not intended to be used as a substitute for a veterinary diagnosis or care. Do not delay seeking proper medical attention based on any advice presented here. The author's intention is to help guide you in recognizing when your pet is having an emergency and to hopefully help get better outcomes (results not guaranteed) by teaching effective techniques in acupressure.

THERE ARE COMMON PET emergencies where acupressure could help you stabilize the patient until you reach your veterinarian. Although I could not list every possible emergency situation, I tried to provide advice in cases where acupressure can help ease pain, calm the pet, and minimize dangerous situations until you can arrive at your veterinarian's office.

Sometimes, as pet owners we get very stressed and panic, having these points information accessible will give something to focus on. Remember that your calmer state of mind will be mimicked by your pet.

PAIN

Stopping pain and suffering is the universal concern of pet owners and veterinarians alike. Painful conditions deemed an emergency require immediate veterinary care.

The way animals demonstrate pain differs, in some cases by a great degree from what humans' experience. This allows for a general misunderstanding of pain in our furry companions. Most people can interpret a dog that is vocalizing or crying from movement or touch as having pain.

Unfortunately, not all dogs are created equal when it comes to pain. There are stoic dogs and super tough guys that do not show any pain. When they do, you better believe their situation is dire. My buddy and super tough police K9 officer Dano ia a good example. His handler noticed he was panting more and seemed reluctant to jump into the patrol car. When I examined him, I noticed proprioceptive deficits in his hind legs, which meant he was dragging his back paws. However, he did not show any pain when I palpated his spine and tried to manipulate him, except looking me in the eye to say stop it and then proceeded to sit down. When I took an x-ray I couldn't believe it. Dano had not one, but three areas in the spine where there were disc issues. I performed acupuncture, put him on some herbs and pain medications and referred him to a neurologist.

Understandably, the Winter Haven Police Department needed to know if he needed to retire from this injury. The neurologist discovered other places where the column was pinched and expressed astonishment as to why this dog was not totally paralyzed or screaming in excruciating pain. Even now as a retired senior dog he is a tough cookie.

Dano taught me a big lesson: do not expect all dogs to show you they are in pain as some are too tough to show any weakness. That realization has come in handy since I've been taking care of the Winter Haven Police Department K-9 Unit for over a decade.

There are other ways that dogs express pain other than crying or panting. Other signs are having leg tremors, not eating, and decreasing their activity level. Most dogs are intuitive. When they hurt, they may not move. Therefore, not wanting to eat is a sign that weighs heavily when evaluating quality of life.

Dogs love to play, interact with their pack, eat, sleep, and repeat the cycle daily. Any deviation from this simple routine should arise the pet owner's suspicion that something is wrong with their pet.

THE FIVE MAIN SIGNS OF PAIN

1. Panting. This could be due to the anxiety they feel at not knowing why they hurt. Dogs that might be feverish, have blood loss anemia, or respiratory distress can also pant. This is usually a pretty good symptom for Cushing's disease, or a hyperactive adrenal. Pain should be the main concern when the panting is exacerbated with exercise or movement.

2. Decreased activity level. This can be subtle. Pay attention to see if your dog is cutting his play time down or avoiding activities like jumping or playing. Remember that dogs and cats love their routines. Whenever you see a deviation from the normal day to day activities, that alone is cause for concern and for a quick visit to your veterinarian.

3. Avoidance. This is your dog telling you he's not playing ball because it hurts to either run, jump, or grab the ball. Oral pain is heavily underestimated and a leading cause of dogs refusing to eat, grab toys, chew hard foods, and grooming themselves.

4. Behavior changes. A dog that is getting grumpy towards you or other furry housemates could be masking pain. I have discovered painful dogs or cats only after they got into big fights with housemates. Upon examination, I've found a myriad of pain causing conditions like abscessed teeth, glaucoma, bladder stones, cancer masses, severe degenerative joint disease, and arthritis. In most cases, cats prefer solitude when in pain; they start hiding more and avoiding interaction with their humans. Cats will miss their

litter boxes and might stop eating if they are in pain. Dogs vary. They might be acting clingier or very aggressive.

5. Crying or vocalizing. If you touch or pick up a sensitive part, an animal may cry, grunt, or growl/hiss in pain. Some pets are truly skittish and will protest anyway, so it's crucial to determine if pain is the cause. Repeat the touch with another person in the household to see if it is a consistent expression. Some senior cats vocalize when they have hallucinations or when they feel threatened, bad, or confused. This could be due to dementia or a disease process like hyperthyroidism.

HELPING YOUR PET IN PAIN

I do not recommend administering human pain medications to pets. The best course of action is to consult your veterinarian or the animal poison control line before even thinking about over-the-counter human medications for your pet. Just one Tylenol will kill your cat or small dog. My heart breaks for all the liver and kidney failures I've seen from people giving aspirin, Aleve, and Tylenol to their pets. Each one was a preventable death where the owners were not malicious, just ignorant about the fatal consequences. All the pain medications out there could be harmful for your pet.

GENERAL ACUPOINTS FOR EMERGENCIES

There are nearly 200 acupoints used in dogs and cats. Pet owners can familiarize themselves with just a few multipurpose, powerful points that can prove useful in cases of common emergencies. Using the tip of your fingers, you can apply firm pressure to these areas. Do not replace acupressure for veterinary care. Please, seek veterinary emergency care as soon as possible.

FOR PAIN CONTROL

Apply firm pressure for one minute, rest and repeat for a total of five times on the following acupoints:

Liv 3- This is a powerful point to move energy blockages. It is on top of the back paw, midway between the second and third finger and feels like a little hole right before a bony ridge (dorsal back paw at the level of the metacarpal fusion of digits 2&3).

Gv20- This is called permission point and has a calming effect. It is in the middle of the top of the head, at the level of the ear canals. Imagine a line across the front and the back of the ear bases. GV20 will be in the middle of those lines and on the midline of the skull.

Gb20- This is a great point for the complementary liver channel which distributes the energy (*Qi*). It is a great for mental issues as well. To find it just simply find the bump at the midline, top back of the skull (occipital ridge) and go off to each side of the neck until you find a little depression. Some colleagues have described how you find this pair of points as "how you pick up a six-pack of beer".

SWELLING

What to do in case of swelling? The adequate treatment varies depending of the cause and location of the swollen area.

Acute swelling could be related to:

» an abscess

» a mass

» an allergic reaction, or

» a traumatic injury.

How can you tell if hot or cold compresses are needed? It depends! The most acute, hot, swollen tissues benefit from a cold compress held to the area for five to ten minutes and on the way to the veterinarian. If you suspect an abscess or a muscle swelling, then a hot compress will do best to draw an opening where the nasty pus could come out.

HIT BY CAR

A common, but unfortunate situation is coming upon an animal that was hit by a car. Regardless whether the victim is your pet or a stray, you must approach with caution. An animal in shock and acute pain is unpredictable. Use a heavy blanket to try to pick up the injured pet. Covering the eyes might help calm the victim. If it is wildlife or a stray, consider calling animal services instead. Try to move the animal minimally, using a blanket as a stretcher might be good, but it won't offer much spine support.

In cases where the animal is semi-comatose, use resuscitation point GV 26. This point is in the midline of the nose, looking at the dog, at the level of the nostrils. Stimulate this point by tapping aggressively on it using a pen or your fingertip. Knowing basic CPR is ideal, but in pets the difference is that chest compressions are extremely important and you don't have to breathe for the pet, just compress.

BREATHING ISSUES

What if the issue is Dyspnea/choking/incessant cough? A cough could mean either a bad heart or lung system as the root problem. There are several excellent acupoints to stop coughs, but the easiest one to reach is CV22. This point is in the tip of the manubrium, or the point where the clavicles meet, right on the front of the chest. Press there firmly for one to three minutes and seek veterinary assistance as soon as possible.

URINATION ISSUES

Difficulty urinating is a very dangerous life or death situation that needs immediate veterinary attention. Cats can have a blockage due to a plug, made out of crystals and sloughed off cells, in their urethra which impedes them to urinate. If the blockage is not relieved within forty-eight hours, the urine back up can hurt the kidneys and the bladder can rupture as well leading to a painful death. Although female cats and dogs get blocked, this awful scenario happens more commonly to males of all species due to a penile urethra that is a lot longer. This is a very urgent situation that requires allopathic medicine intervention as soon as possible.

However, after the crisis, in order to prevent a recurrence, you can

» Do daily *tui na* massage

» Provide special supplements containing D-mannose (a derivative from cranberries) and vitamin C

» Encourage your pet to drink a lots of water

» Feed them mainly canned pet food

The owners can try easing the pain and inflammation by doing acupressure on Liv3 to control the pain while on way to veterinary care. This point was described previously. Adding pressure on a point strictly used for bladder is even better. An accessible point is called Bl 39 and is found on the back of the knee, on the lateral (outside side) of back skin crease of the knee. The precise anatomical description says is lies on the inside of the Biceps femoris tendon at the level of the crease. Put acupressure there while you transport to your veterinarian. It is a great point to acupressure after urinary tract surgery and may speed the recovery process.

VOMITING/DIARRHEA

The main thing to do is rest the GI tract by stopping all food and water for a minimum of twelve hours. The points CV 8 and CV 12 will help ease the belly pain. You will find these points located in the ventral midline, or underside of the pet. CV8 corresponds to the umbilicus. Rub in a circular firm pattern right at the umbilicus and follow the imaginary midline all the way to the sternum, where the ribs meet in the underside. It marks the chest area by slightly protruding and feels like a soft bone, but is cartilage. Massage with the palm of the hand creating friction and warmth. Go back and forth several times. The CV12 is located midway between the umbilicus and the sternum and is considered the alarm point for stomach issues. If you rub your pet there and he flinches or shows pain, that pet has a stomach issue. This could be stomach ulcers, parasites, early bloat, foreign objects causing trouble, or just pure food indigestion. Although this point is useful to localize the pain and diagnose, it also helps in treating. For example, gentle daily massage helps pets with chronic acid reflux.

ANAPHYLAXIS

Allergic reactions are widely varied, but mostly show as swelling around the head, hives, or rashes. Cooling compresses and topical Benadryl creams might help until you get vet assistance. Acupressure on GV 14 might be very helpful too. You find this point in the front of your pet's scapulas, dorsally, on the imaginary top of their body's midline. You could move up the neck and wherever it stops bending and meets the trunk of the body, that's the point.

Toxins can be absorbed orally or through the skin. If the toxic chemicals are in skin, wash the area with baby shampoo or hand soap and rinse thoroughly. If the toxin was ingested, collect the containers to take with you to the vet's office and press on Liv3 on the way there.

SEIZURES

Another scary situation for pet owners is witnessing their furry friend having a seizure. As horrible as it looks, seizures can be managed and your pet can have a great quality of life. Traditional Chinese Veterinary Medicine (TCVM) offers a new way to manage seizures. In TCVM, the seizures are associated with a disorder in the Liver, Kidney, Heart, and Spleen TCVM organs. Seizures can be caused by many underlying patterns. The main course of action is to make sure the pet is not in a bed, a place where it can fall down, or near a pool where it could accidentally fall and drown.

The owners can apply acupressure on An Shen, GV 20, or GB 20 until they can seek veterinary help. An Shen works for anxiety and compulsive disorders. You find this point past GB20, directly on the back of the ears. Feel the fossa there and apply firm pressure.

Some of my clients like to use essential oils, especially lavender, for seizure control. My advice is to dilute the essential oil by placing a couple of drops in a small amount of coconut oil and apply to the acupoints described above.

Please try to notice how long the seizure lasts and what your pet is doing while it is occurring. Your veterinarian needs as much information as you can provide in order to gauge what kind of treatment is needed. I have included more information about TCVM treatment of seizures in the healing with herbs chapter.

When it comes to emergency situations, TCVM can be of great assistance, but your ultimate goal must be to seek veterinary emergency care as soon as possible. As I previously mentioned, Allopathic medicine shines for acute issues whereas TCVM's strength is in managing chronic disease processes. The ultimate approach is integrated medicine in which both work in tandem to the benefit of your pets.

CHAPTER 10

FINDING THE LONGEVITY SOLUTION

•   •   •   •

"AN OUNCE OF PREVENTION it is worth a pound of cure," is a saying that I take very seriously. Holistic pet care means that we are looking at the animal as a whole and taking care of not just their physical needs, but mental needs as well. It also means looking at the environment, behavior, and the human animal bond. I know that you are likely reading this book because you care deeply about your pet's well-being and want your companion to live a long and healthy life.

If people were more like their pets, then the world would be a much better place. Our companion animals give us unconditional love and support. To them we are the best regardless of how we look, what our bank balance is, or how we are feeling that day. Pets live in the moment; they enjoy each day while they show love to their owners and honestly express how they feel. Therefore, we must think about prevention medicine as a means to increase the time we get to share with our companions.

My ideal plan for your pet includes exercise, nutrition, twice a year veterinary checkups, dental care, grooming, socialization, and obedience training (for dogs). Alternative medicine modalities like food therapy, acupuncture, herbals, and massage can be seamlessly integrated to help keep your pet in optimal health. This plan is the key to finding the longevity solution to maximize your pet's health to increase their lifespan naturally.

Exercise and mental stimulation for your companion pet

When it comes to exercise, you must remember that physical activity is an integral part of any wild animal's day to day existence. How does that relate to our seemingly couch potato pets?

Let's start with man's best friend. Your dog's ancestors are closely related to the Grey Wolf. Wolves roam large territories looking for food, working as a pack, and are extremely intelligent. It was through domestication and association with ancient humans that a bond exists today between humans and dogs. In modern society, we tend to forget that dogs need a good deal of mental stimulation and exercise. There is more to it than just the physical benefits of being fit and strong. The energy that dogs have needs to be spent or it will result in poor health, obesity, and severe behavioral disorders.

Walking with your dogs on a daily basis is the single most important thing that you can do to establish a deep connection with them. In their eyes, you are the alpha and when you walk them you are establishing your role. Of course, first you must learn how to walk them properly. They should be at your side, never pulling you forward. Ideally they should stop when you stop and be trained to look at your face to seek approval of their actions before doing them.

The importance of the exercise routine is the physical challenge that a long walk presents for both you and your dog. Each will benefit tremendously because you will burn some extra calories while lessening the damage that comes with overfeeding your animals. There is an epidemic of obesity in this country and it extends to the animals. I have seen a big rise in obesity in our dogs, cats, and even small mammals kept as pets.

I took care of one Chihuahua that was supposed to weigh under five to six pounds. He weighed a whopping eight pounds. He was lethargic and we ran blood work to find out if there was an underlying reason for the obesity issue other than overfeeding table scraps and cheap dog food. His blood sugar was slightly high and this was a wakeup call for his owners. I presented the options: (1) A lifelong administration of insulin or (2) change the diet by cutting the pizza, cheese, and other junky treats out while increasing the amount of exercise. The owners began to walk him and changed his diet and, within a couple months, this little Chihuahua had lost one pound. The extra benefits included better mobility and for the most part he was less stiff getting up and down. He had luxated patellas (knee caps), a congenital condition that results in weak knees and usually causes severe arthritis in middle aged and senior dogs. Another surprising side effect of shedding the extra weight was that his usual grumpy demeanor had improved. This told me he really might have been experiencing some pain related to the pressure of the extra pounds on those weak knees.

UNDERLYING METABOLISM ISSUES

In some cases of obese dogs, I have discovered an underlying reason causing their metabolism to function poorly. Take for example a sweet Shih Tzu named Sunny. He first came to us because he could not walk due to a slipped disk. Even though I did not perform acupuncture at the time, we still got him over the paralysis by offering nutraceuticals, a small course of steroids, and physical rehab. He was a chubby dog and we stressed the importance of losing the extra pounds to prevent another back issue. The owner swore she was feeding a high quality food and the amounts seemed reasonable. Luckily, we checked his body enzyme functions and to our surprise, his thyroid hormone was very low. The thyroid is the hormone that, among many functions, controls the metabolic rate of your pet's body. Sunny started supplementation with the thyroid hormone and extended his daily walks. He promptly lost the excess weight. That was almost a decade ago and he never had another issue with his back. He suffers from arthritis on his front legs, but gets relief with regular acupuncture and massage therapy. He is a living example of how a committed owner can help their pet's lose the weight and live a much better life.

The basic rule to lose weight remains the same: calories in, calories out. If we burn more calories than we consume, we will experience weight loss. No magic pills, no fancy cures and the same applies for our furry friends. The good thing is that unlike us, our pets cannot open the refrigerator to eat whatever they want, whenever they want it. We are in control of how much they eat and should take the responsibility seriously. Obesity is a big factor that contributes to heart disease, diabetes, thyroid disease, and arthritis.

HEALTHY WEIGHT CAN ADD YEARS TO YOUR PET'S LIFE

There was a big lifespan study made by Purina that lasted from 1987 until 2002. It concluded that when you restrict the calories and keep the dogs at ideal weight, not only will they live 15% longer, but in their senior years they will have less symptoms of arthritis. The Labradors on that study averaged two extra years. In other words, not only will your dog be able to live longer, but it will have less arthritic pain and enjoy a better quality of life longer than an obese dog. If that doesn't motivate you to hit the trail with your pet, I don't know what will! Cats also suffer from an obesity epidemic. Thankfully, exercising your cat is very simple. Some people use harnesses to train their cats to walk outside just like they would a dog. Even if you're not willing to try that technique, there are simpler ways to accomplish the same results. First, you can buy a laser light pointer or the fishing rod type toy. You can also just use a string and plain paper bags to provide your cat with the fun and games to actually run around the house. Restricting the amount of calories they consume will help tremendously.

Diabetes in cats is an extremely common consequence of being obese. I remember one patient Tony, a big tomcat that was urinating all over the house and drinking lots of water. The owner was devastated when I diagnosed him with Diabetes. She preferred holistic medicine and dreaded using insulin. Her sweet Tony turned into a tiger whenever he needed to be medicated. She asked me if we could reverse the Diabetes. I told her that cats are very special animals and Diabetes is almost always a lifestyle disease that could be reversed by making dramatic feeding changes.

We used an herbal formula called Ophiopogon and changed his diet to a medicated commercial diet for Diabetes. The diet is high protein and low carbs which helps to control the blood sugar levels. The owner bought a laser pen and started forcing him to exercise at home. As the excess pounds were shed, we also noticed a downward trend in his sugar numbers. We never gave him insulin, yet his Diabetes went into remission within six months of the new changes. He is an elderly cat now and still looks half his age.

When it comes to the amount of food to give your pet, do not follow the recommendations on the food bag blindly. Those recommendations tend to feed large quantities because they do not take into account the sedentary lifestyle of your pets. Your holistic veterinarian can prepare a homemade diet specific to your pet's condition. Food therapy using the proper energetic qualities of the food items to address disease processes and prevention has been proven to save many pets and extend their quality of life. Although there are no acupoints to lose weight, there are acupoints to increase endurance and energy that may be appropriate in your natural weight loss regimen.

My advice is to always ask your veterinarian which amount of food is appropriate. The best trick to know if your pet is in great shape is to feel the ribs. If you can see the ribs on the dog or cat, they are too skinny. If you can feel the top of the ribs, but you do not feel any indentations in between the ribs that is ideal weight. If you cannot feel the individual ribs or the top of the ribs, your pet is officially a meatball!Also, remember to count treats as food. Lots of owners cut down on the food, but then give either an excessive number of treats or a small number of calorie rich junky ones. Treats do have a lot of calories and these add up. Cut the treats and use small amounts of lean meats or veggies instead of store bought ones.

HOW MUCH EXERCISE?

How much exercise is *too* much? One could definitely overdo it, especially in elderly or arthritic dogs, or pets that have cardiac conditions. Before you start your new exercise program, take your pet to the veterinarian for a good checkup and discuss your plan of action. Get the official "OK" and feel good that you are doing what's best for your pet. In very arthritic dogs, acupuncture can help control pain and a moderate exercise regimen can then be started.

How does exercise help the mental health of our pets? Exercise releases endorphins and makes you feel great, so one could assume it does the same for your pets. That's not all though. It provides vital mental stimulation essential for pets. Dogs and cats possess an olfactory part of the brain that is large compared to humans'. They derive much pleasure from smelling different scents. Everything they see during your walks serves as mental stimulation and an outlet for the energy they possess. If in the wild they would normally hunt up to ten hours a day and now you come along and solve that issue by providing their food, then what do they do with the rest of the day? If they achieve their main objective by eating so quickly and so frequently, there must be something else to engage their energy with. How long do you need to exercise them then? I recommend dog owners to at least walk them for half an hour twice a day. Cats I reccomend ten minutes twice a day if you want them to lose weight and at least five minutes twice a day for maintenance.

Foraging and exercise needs can be met concurrently by using interactive toys specific for each species. For example, if you have pet birds, you should purchase interactive pet toys or make them yourself to try to encourage foraging. Exotic pets need to work for food. Hide the food or change the places where you feed them every day. These simple changes can really impact their mental health and stimulate the part of the brain that figures out puzzles. Same applies to cats; change the feeding places, use toys that release treats if they perform an action, or make them exercise before you feed them. You will find more cooperation for your obedience training and for any training in general if your pet is a little hungry.

You can use food as a powerful exercise and foraging motivator and as a positive reward. If you overfeed your pet, he or she will most likely become overweight and refuse to exercise.

Birds and exotics need big enough enclosures and different perches or hiding places depending on the species. The best strategy here is to recreate their natural habitat as much as you can and you will have a happier exotic pet. Do your research before you buy any exotic pet and ask your veterinarian for species specific advice on their care.

The holistic view is that health is the balance between body and mind. Some people might argue that pets do not need mental and emotional care, but I wholeheartedly disagree. All animals, especially exotics, need mental stimulation and enrichment.

Many acupoints can be used to treat self-inflicted injuries such as feather picking, fur pulling, chewing tails, etc. Most of these issues have the root cause in a lack of proper husbandry and environmental enrichment. It is best to address the underlying causes before attempting any treatment.

FOOD MATTERS

I consider feeding a high-quality diet, appropriate to the life stage and species of your pet, one of the best investments that you can make. Providing the right food is the main way of supplying the necessary energy to heal and to maintain optimal health in your pet's body. If you give poor food, you will get poor health results.

When it comes to feeding, quantity is just as important as quality, so make sure to use a measuring cup when providing dry kibble. Take into consideration everything your pet gets during the day like regular feedings, treats, treats, and more treats. The calories keep accumulating so try to look for more natural treats such as fresh meat, carrots, or even broccoli stalks. It is best to stay away from fatty, processed snacks from the table for most part. If you follow these suggestions, you will begin to start seeing the difference in short order.In the Food Therapy chapter, I went into extensive detail about the energetics and value of certain foodstuffs. It should be adequate it to say that a high-quality diet should be an integral part of any wellness plan for your pet. If you have any exotic pets, this is critical. Many of the diseases that I see in birds and pocket pets are related to inadequate husbandry practices. Research the natural diet of your exotic pet and try to keep as close to it as you can. Failure to provide the proper nutrition will impede your pet's ability to thrive and will shorten their lifespan.

CALCIUM FOR REPTILES AND BIRDS

An improperly supplemented diet will result in a pet that looks lethargic and may even develop bone fractures. It is very sad to see iguanas and bearded dragons that come in sick and weak due to poor husbandry. I have taken many x-rays of iguanas where the outline of each bone is barely visible. Their diets were so low in calcium that the body had no other recourse than to absorb calcium from the bones to survive. Even when pet owners fed enough calcium, they may fail to provide enough ultraviolet light for the reptiles to be able to absorb that calcium.

I have reversed many of these cases, but unfortunately there is a point that many will die regardless of treatment. Calcium is an essential nutrient across the board for all species. I have seen reptiles that have dramatic outward signs of vitamin and mineral deficiencies. For example, tortoises and turtle shells will be completely deformed when lacking certain vitamins such as A and D. In some reptiles, the bones will bend just like rubber bands and multiple fractures may be detected fairly easily.

I have also seen many pet reptiles come in refusing to eat. As soon as the right food with the right environment is provided, they will start eating. Live prey is better for most carnivorous reptiles, as they receive mental stimulation when trying to catch their food and thrive better than when being fed canned or frozen diets. Exotic pets can live multiple decades if housed and fed properly.

FOOD ALLERGIES

There are many external signs of disease caused by inadequate. In my hospital, I have found a direct link between food allergies and chronic ear and skin issues. I meet many allergic dogs that are miserable and itchy for years. Most of these pets' owners have considered euthanizing them due to their poor quality of life.

I remember a Border Collie that had been given steroid injections to control her constant itching. I could not finish my examination because she was constantly scratching. The owner had her on a low-cost, chicken-based diet. I told her to switch to a better quality lamb diet and treated her with acupuncture and herbs. Imagine my delight when my client said she slept through the night after her first session. Weeks later, the owner ran out of the new food. So she decided to temporarily go back to the old diet. Unfortunately for her Border Collie, this started the itch-scratch cycle all over again. That experience convinced her that the diet was an integral part of her dog's skin health and her quality of life was immediately improved by a simple change in food.

Many allergic dogs live shorter lives due to the chronic use of steroids and other stronger pharmaceuticals that may cause side effects and organ failure. In a study published in 1997, the effects of steroids in mice was studied and measured. They concluded that 87% of the mice given steroids died earlier than their lifespan. Only 12% of the control group died earlier than expected. Of those mice that died using steroids, the autopsy revealed disease which included tumors in the liver, kidneys, and heart. This indicates to me that a simple food trial or a food allergy test can be a lifesaver for many dogs and cats suffering from food allergies.

Acupuncture can be used to control pain and to treat many conditions without damaging side effects. Along with herbals and food therapy, a long term care plan can be developed that will spare the major organs and provide a longer lifespan despite chronic disease.

There are also inward signs of disease that can only be found after performing a blood panel. Some dogs, ferrets, and cats come in my office with seizures or in a coma because their blood sugar is too low. Other patients are examples of how too much and too rich a diet can cause diabetes and other health issues. The power of food is such that it can basically heal or kill you. This is why I always recommend investing in high-quality food for your pet. In addition, I suggest using supplements wisely and utilizing all the holistic benefits of food as advised by your veterinarian. This approach is a proven way to increase the lifespan of your companion pets.

FREQUENT VETERINARY VISITS PAY OFF

I am a firm advocate of twice a year veterinary checkups. Animal bodies deteriorate at a much faster rate than humans do so it's crucial for these checkups. Many people think that dogs age at a rate of seven years for each human year, but that is not true. Dogs and cats go into teenage years or childbearing age pretty quickly. So in most cases, the first year could be equal to twelve or fifteen years of a human's life. Depending on the weight and species, the animals will age at a different rate. In dogs, smaller breeds deteriorate at a rate average of four years versus seven to a big giant breed. This concept of body deterioration supports my recommendation of getting your pet thoroughly examined by a veterinarian at least twice a year.

Imagine if you only went to the doctor every four years. Think of how many health issues will accrue and cause additional problems. I recommend a full-blood panel yearly to determine the inner health and to screen for potential problems prior to the appearance of any clinical signs of disease. A proactive approach allows me to treat conditions earlier. This means a higher chance to turn things around for the better by intervening and either switching diets, changing lifestyles, and/or starting supplementation with herbal therapy. Twice a year exams are great opportunities for you and your veterinarian to talk about wellness goals or any concerns you might have with your pet.Experts working with one of the largest corporate chain of veterinary offices, conducted a mega study on pet lifespans. The data was collected from two million dogs and almost a half million cats seen at their offices. They concluded that the average lifespan of cats and dogs has increased by at least one year nationwide. They credit their twice a year veterinary visit protocol and preventive medicine with that increase in longevity. I see my patients living longer also. They have better lives since I started advising them to come at least twice a year.

I have several senior pets with perfect results in their blood panels. When they come in for their six month checkup, we make sure repeat the lab work. Sometimes they sometimes show symptoms of organ disease. One of those was a Papillon that belongs to my practice manager. He had lost a half pound and seemed to start urinating more, but was otherwise fine. We checked him every six months to monitor a heart murmur and his Cushing's disease. The owner was concerned, so we repeated the blood tests earlier. To our surprise, he was a full blown diabetic. We were able to find out in time to save his eyesight and to avoid lasting organ damage. I used acupuncture, herbs, and insulin to restore his health. His case showed all my technicians and veterinary associates how important frequent examinations and blood-work truly are.

PETS WANT TO SMILE TOO

Another integral part of any wellness plan for your pets is dental care. Even the most holistic doctors agree that dental disease affects the whole body in multiple ways. Billions of bacteria form plaque in the teeth that continuously invade your pet's bloodstream where they can reach the heart. The American Animal Hospital Association (AAHA) has cited studies that reveal that nearly 70% of pet owners do not provide the dental care recommended by veterinarians. They recognized dental disease links to heart and organ disease and because of the health impact of these on all pets, they developed the comprehensive *AAHA's Dental Care Guidelines for Dogs and Cats* (updated in 2013).

In a few cases, clients have come to me for holistic and natural care of their pets, but do not want to take care of obvious periodontal and dental disease issues. I can use acupuncture to strengthen the Kidney channel (which controls the teeth), to relieve dental pain, and also to tonify the Spleen channel (which controls the gums). I can recommend a good diet that would get the heat (inflammation) out of the mouth and treats that can help scrape some of the tartar off. However, I must recommend a complete oral assessment under light sedation whenever possible because it is the most effective way to restore a painful, diseased mouth to proper health. Technological advances in patient monitoring, digital radiography, and safer anesthesia makes treatment of dental disease a sound investment in your pet's health.

I remember the case of a very grumpy and obese small dog that had horrible dental disease. He came in because his face was swollen and the owner thought he had been stung by a bee or was sick. It turns out that one of his teeth was so infected that the root caused an abscess that broke through the skin and into the eye. Sadly, this is a common occurrence and also completely preventable. Many dogs that come into our practice with a tooth abscesses can have a favorable outcome. We remove the rotten tooth, flush the area, put bone implant material into the empty socket, and close the defect. They recover quickly and the owners realize how much pain the pets were in after they see them acting peppier and happier after their procedure.

Did you know obesity can be a sign of a painful teeth? Affected dogs and cats will swallow dry food, but will not chew their food. They end up eating a lot more because the act of chewing is the starting point of digestion. Lots of whole kibble gets eaten, but because they are not being predigested with the salivary enzymes, nutrients might not be well absorbed and the signal of satiety to the brain is delayed.

Other pets come to me for chronic issues of vomiting and diarrhea along with picky eating. A majority of these cases also have advanced dental disease.

An extreme example of dental disease causing harm to a pet's health was a small dog that came to us for a behavior consultation and evaluation. The dog began attacking his owner and trying to bite people and other dogs. He was a senior, three pound Pomeranian full of rage. When I examined him, I noticed a rotting smell from his mouth. A quick peek under his lips revealed green teeth that were moving like piano keys. I explained to my client that her dog had a very severe mouth infection and oral pain. In fact, he had all forty-two teeth extracted due to the advanced periodontal disease. Within days after his dental surgery, the owner informed us that his behavior issue was almost completely resolved. I believe he will live longer and better just by taking care of that severe infection and painful condition.

I have many clients worried about the anesthesia risks during dental procedures. Even the most resistant owners can tell you that after we intervened, cleaned the teeth, and took care of all the diseased teeth, their pet's general attitude and health improved dramatically. You have to realize that your dog's and cat's rotten teeth can extend into their sinuses because that is where the roots usually end. A rotten tooth root can interfere with your pet's amazing ability to smell, curtailing their enjoyment of the world around them.

Pet owners must have some kind of home care plan for their pet's teeth. Imagine what would happen to your mouth if you did not floss or brush your teeth on a daily basis. In some aspects, your dog or cat is like a tiny person with a furry coat on and they deserve good dental hygiene and care. Providing this care will allow them to live longer.

LOOKING GOOD

When it comes to grooming your pet, do not think that this is a vanity affair. We are not just talking about making your pet look good, it is about making sure that basic hygiene and maintenance procedures are being taken care of. This makes your pet feel better and prevents certain disease processes from wreaking havoc in your pet's coat.

The minimum coat care dogs and cats need is a daily brushing. This can be a bonding experience for you and your pets. It's also a great way of lowering your blood pressure since it can place you in a sort of meditative state. Daily brushing prevents matted fur, which is the culprit of many skin infections and it very painful to your pet. The skin underneath the mats is where infections can flourish.Excessive shedding could be a sign of the season or that you need to brush your pet more often. Flat faced breeds have many skin folds that can easily get infected, especially during the hot summer days. Another good practice is clipping the sanitary trail, around the genitals and anus, of your pets. This is done to facilitate urination and defecation by preventing excrement and urine to stick to the fur. Also, on hairy breeds, cleaning around the eyes and plucking the ear hair will prevent infections, whereas clipping the underneath of the paws and trimming the nails can help them with proper gait and posture.

A healthy pet will have a luxurious coat. After all, the skin is the largest organ. Acupuncture and customized diets will help animals suffering from chronic skin issues, but the owners must also practice basic grooming to keep the coat healthier.

What kind of health issues can be linked to the state of the fur in our pets? When I see greasy or matted fur, I immediately suspect the pet is not healthy. Oftentimes, a greasy coat means the pet is too sick to self-groom. Perhaps they are grooming, but because they have periodontal disease, the stinky saliva makes the fur appear oily. A dry and scaly coat could reveal the pet has anemia, a vitamin deficiency, or even parasites. Changes in coat color, like a bleached appearance or darkening, could mean there are underlying hormonal deficiencies like Hypothyroidism. Small hairless spots could actually be skin tumors, so any concerning changes in your pet's coat could potentially mean a shorter lifespan if not taken care of medically.

CHOOSING THE RIGHT PET

Cats

Choosing the right kind of pet for your lifestyle will go a long ways to ensure that pets are well taking care of and they match your available time for interaction. A well matched owner and pet will develop a stronger bond that assures that mutual enjoyment and satisfaction.

For busy animal lovers, the best companion is a cat.

I love cats because I feel so attuned with their curious and independent demeanor. The truth is, you cannot buy the affection of a cat. When they freely express their love and approval, it makes me feel fantastic. Cats are solitary animals, but they will form small groups and express social behavior. That makes them great for apartment dwellers and owners that work long hours.

Many people may argue that they have multiple cats and they all get along. I agree; I've had up to five felines at a time without any major issues. I'm not saying that they don't want other cat's company, but I believe they do not need a pack to be fulfilled.

I grew up with cats as my confidants and friends. I spent many hours observing their behavior and interactions. I can tell you that cats can live by themselves with no detriment to their mental health as long as they have a good bond with their owner and their environment provides them with stimulating activities.

Cats often tolerate one another. Cats are very territorial; they will claim sections of the house where each cat will have their domain and congregate in areas of neutral territory, where group activities like eating and grooming can happen. This territorialism usually extends to guarding resources, which is the main reason I advise having one more litter box than the number of cats living in a household.

Adopting an older cat is great since their personality and behavior is set. Most people want to adopt kittens which are adorable. Look how many Youtube ™ videos have been made about them. All kittens are rambunctious until about a year of age because their personalities are not yet set. Many pet owners try to bypass this wild stage by declawing their babies. I oppose doing this painful amputation of their paws because it has zero medical benefit and it actually increases chances of behavioral problems, like urinating or defecating out of the litter box. As a result, they often end up biting more.

The CDC and NIH have both stated that declawing cats is not recommended if you are immune-suppressed. The reason is that cats becoming more prone to biting. You may be surprised to know that Cat Scratch Fever is more likely to be transmitted by a cat bite than a scratch. Many declawed cats have complications and earlier onset of polyarthritis as a consequence of declawing. Even with aggressive pain control, this is still a painful procedure. Some argue that surgery with a laser is much safer and painless. Unfortunately, that has no bearing on the long-term consequences of amputating the toes. This procedure often alters the cat's gait, may cause the rest of digits' joints to fuse, and can be chronically painful. I believe declawing a cat could shorten his or her lifespan because the arthritis pain could be a quality of life factor and some people might decide to euthanize earlier.

After two decades in practice, I decided to follow the advice of fellow veterinarian Jennifer Conrad and abandoned this procedure altogether. I now encourage all cat owners to visit www.thepawproject.org to learn more about this issue and make a compassionate decision. In 2015, I joined a nationwide group of conscientious veterinarians that offer repair surgery for botched declawed cats in need of pain relief.

How can you avoid the destruction of your property by cat claws? All kittens need scratching posts that are sturdy and that offer different scratching experiences. Some cats like scratching horizontal surfaces and some prefer vertical ones. Some like the cardboard texture and other the rope; it's all about watching what they prefer and offering those. Put catnip on those scratching posts or spray with pheromones like Feliway ™ spray.

There are many ways to discourage furniture destruction like using saran wrap or crinkly materials over your furniture until they learn to avoid them. Clipping the nails regularly, every three weeks, will help too. In my house, we used plastic water pistols placed all around the living areas and easily accessible by anyone witnessing any of my kitties trying to claw the furniture or climb on counters. A small squirt of water makes them stop the behavior immediately. The best thing is they do not associate that correction with us.

There is an ingenious invention called Soft Paws ™ that covers the nail with a plastic cap glued to it. It is a very simple solution to the destructive nature of the nails and it is easier to start all kittens and continue until adulthood. Not to mention that the nails come in all fun colors and make your cat look very fashionable.

Dogs

On the other end of the spectrum, we have dogs. Dogs are pack animals and many times they need another dog to fulfill themselves. I am not criticizing single dog homes but it is definitely easier for a dog to learn and be trained when they have role models of their same kind in the household. Cats might do very well without much interaction, but dogs want a lot more of their human's attention. For very busy business people then, they need to look at their lifestyle and think twice before they decide to share their lives with a dog. The owners of single dogs must provide socialization and dog to dog interaction opportunities such as daycare, dog walking groups, playdates, etc.

Puppies present a lot of challenges for the novice pet owner. They explore the world with their mouths so you must toddler proof your house and prepare to supervise them at all times. They need veterinary care and lots of socialization. Their first year could be very expensive, but the steps you take to neuter/spay, vaccinate, socialize, and train will last a lifetime of health. The Banfield Pet study published in 2013 says that spay and neutering cats and dogs does increase their lifespan.

I do not recommend ear cropping for the same reason I am against declawing: no medical benefit.

Your puppy looks up to you to follow your lead on how to behave so make sure you do the reading and research into your dog's breed and general care they'll need. Be the leader of the pack early on. They will learn faster if they can model after older dogs in the households. I truly recommend you invest in professional obedience classes and prepare to be patient. Knowing where the puppy comes from is important because temperament is hereditary. The old adage of "the apple doesn't fall far from the tree" is true. Your veterinarian is a great source of advice so choose a practice that has behavior counseling, daycare, and obedience classes available to guide and help you shape your puppy.

Whatever time you invest to educate your new puppy you will have a return ten times bigger. Some breeds are a bit more stubborn to train, and some rescued puppies come with behavioral issues that may require help from an animal behaviorist. Not all dogs are created equal; some dog breeds have been developed for hunting, herding, or companionship. If you choose a herding dog and you work all day and live in a small apartment, you are setting yourself up for failure! That highly energetic herding dog will develop ways to express that energy that will not agree with your expectations. In other words, they become destructive, anxious, and true behavioral nightmares.

Where you get your dog from also matters. I support adoption for the obvious reason that we have an ongoing pet overpopulation crisis in the U.S. However, I also understand the draw of a certain breed that shares characteristics you seek in a furry companion. I love German Shepherds; I have had most as rescues, but have also purchased two of them. If you are going to buy, I would research the right breeder, interview their methods, and visit them often. For example, the breeders of service dogs have carefully selected their sires and dams for certain temperament, intelligence, and adaptability, which is crucial for these working dogs. If you buy a service dog puppy, the breeder should show you how many of these dogs have made it to being a highly trained companion.

There are many purebred rescue organizations with seniors and puppies available for adoption and ready for a second chance. Before you choose to purchase, check these rescues first, you might be surprised.

If you decide to adopt a puppy from a shelter, it is important to understand that many pets there carry emotional baggage and may need time to learn to trust again. Earlier in my career, I worked with the Humane Society on animal cruelty investigations and witnessed the extreme resilience and capacity of abused animals to adapt and overcome. Understanding Dog Behavior

One of the main reasons animals end up in shelters is due to behavioral issues. About 90% of them are completely avoidable if the pet owners would choose the right pet for their lifestyle.

In my practice, we are lucky to have animal behaviorist and international Agility competitor Marco Magiolo to assist all new owners with their companions. One of the cases we had was Lacey, a very aggressive dog that came for a behavioral consult. The owner was frustrated and near her breaking point because Lacey was so aggressive toward other dogs that she could not even walk her or have visitors without being concerned she would attack them. Marco began behavior modification exercises and noticed that Lacey needed socialization. He recommended agility training to burn the excess energy and consulted with me to prescribe a calming herbal formula called Shen calmer "Shen=Mind". It was not easy, but with behavior modification Lacey learned that other dogs were not a threat. Marco enrolled her in daycare and she is now a fun, play-loving, sweet part of our daycare dog pack.

In that case, a holistic approach based on behavior modification, exercise, agility, daycare, and herbals helped save this dog's life and brought closeness and enjoyment to her human owner.

Another similar case was that of Loki the Shetland Shepherd, who came to see Marco because he was destroying everything at home. Loki was an ultra-hyperactive and energetic dog. Unfortunately, her owner's life situation made it difficult to spend much quality time with him. She worked as a bus driver and her schedule was so unpredictable, she would sometimes wake up at three am to arrive on time for her job.

After a previous examination on Loki, we enrolled him in agility classes and daycare. The change in his behavior was nothing short of a miracle according to the owner. Loki was destroying everything at home because he had a lot of energy and was bored. He is an example of how a very energetic dog can recover and be happy even with a busy owner.

Owning a pet is an awesome responsibility. You should explore all alternatives before giving up on your dog's behavior.

My message to all new pet owners is to be patient with puppies and kittens and to take a chance on an adult rescued pet. Your pet is not going to be perfect all the time, he or she will make mistakes and will try your patience on a few occasions. With love and understanding of your dog's shortcomings though, you can really enjoy a deep bond with your pet. Obedience training is mainly a class for the pet owners since most behavioral issues are caused by the way we treat our pets. If we do not learn how to react properly, i.e. when to reward their behavior and when to correct them, there is no chance to change them for the better. Sadly, many pets will suffer abandonment and die early and needlessly. The time and effort you put into your furry friends may very well save their lives.

FINAL THOUGHTS

• • • •

IN EARLY 2016, THE UNIVERSITY of Washington launched the dog aging study, focusing on the effects of a drug called Rapamycin on thousands of dog's lifespans. We cannot stop or slow down aging with a magic pill; it is going to take a multimodal approach to increase the longevity and quality of your pet's life.

Even if your pet is already suffering from a disease condition or is a senior citizen, you can maximize the time you have with your pet by adopting a holistic perspective. Start seeing your pet's health as a puzzle comprised of many pieces such as nutrition, mental stimulation, exercise, veterinary care, and dental health.

You can influence the quality of life of your pet by being involved in their health care. Alternative medicine options are there to help you manage and prevent disease using more natural methods with less damaging side effects. As new doctors, we take the Hippocratic Oath: First do no harm. Acupuncture, Herbal, Food and Massage Therapy, used appropriately, will help your pets without harming them. Adopting a holistic medical approach will add invaluable years with your faithful companions.

APPENDIX A

TIPS FOR HEALING AND WELLNESS OF YOUR PET

• • • •

THIS APPENDIX CONTAINS SIMPLE recipes for a variety of different pets that are easy to prepare in the kitchen.

Marrow broth for Cancer or Critically Ill pets

Bones from a whole chicken or sliced beef bones (oxtails will do)

1- tablespoon vinegar or lemon juice

1 cup carrots chopped

1 cup celery chopped

1 cup kale or spinach chopped

1 cup beets cubed

1 cup shiitake mushrooms

1 tablespoon of Turmeric powder

Place bones in a soup pot or crock pot. Fill with water to cover the bones. Add vegetables, vinegar (or lemon juice). Bring to a boil, then reduce heat to low and simmer for 4-8 hours. More water can be added as needed. Remove the bones and strain the vegetables out at the end. This nutrient rich broth can be given in small frequent servings to anorexic or debilitated cats and dogs. The simple ingredients are easy to digest. This soup will gel in the refrigerator, which is normal.

Dudley's Liver Disease Diet

5 Boneless/skinless chicken breasts (cubed) OR 2 packages of firm tofu cubed

4 oz Sesame oil

8 oz Light soy sauce

2 Tbsp Ginger root, finely grated

6 Tbsp Garlic, crushed

(marinate 20 minutes)

4 Tbsp Canola oil

2 C Cashews, chopped

1lb Green beans, cut

1 C chicken broth

4 Tbsp Corn starch

7 C Brown rice, cooked

1lb Lentils (cooked)

5-6 Sweet potatoes (mashed)

Marinate chicken for 20 minutes. Heat wok to medium high. Add canola oil to wok, stir fry chicken mixture 5-7 minutes. Add cashews and cook for 2 minutes. Add green beans and continue cooking for 4-5 minutes. Mix cornstarch into chicken broth is a separate dish until cornstarch is dissolved, add to wok. Heat thoroughly. Remove from heat and add remaining ingredients, stir until combined. Let cool and separate into individual serving. Feed one cup per 10 lbs of body weight. Store in refrigerator.

Weak and Anorexic Patient

3 cups water

1 pound lean ground beef

1 pound ground chicken

1 cup dry mung beans

1 cup dry barley

¼ cup molasses

2 tablespoons Olive Oil

8oz mushrooms

2 celery stalks, chopped

1 sweet potato, chopped into cubes

1 yellow squash, chopped

Combine all ingredients into a large crock pot. Cook on low for 5-8 hours until lentils are soft and water is absorbed. Feed 1 cup for every 10 pounds of body weight. Adjust serving size according to individual's needs.

**Add to food, just before serving:

Bone Meal 1 teaspoon

½ teaspoon dry mustard

½ teaspoon marjoram

1 garlic cloves, finely chopped

No Guilt Ice Cream

3 medium frozen bananas

5 capsules of probiotics

1 tbsp vanilla

3 tbsp peanut or almond butter

3 tbsp honey

Combine in your food processor and serve. You might portion out in ice tray and refreeze or enjoy it yourself.

Mung Bean Soup

For pets with Liver disease, stomach ulcers, heat rashes or autoimmune blood disease mung bean soup could help their body in releasing the excess heat produced by those inflammatory conditions. You will need;

2 cups of Mung beans

6-8 cups of water

2 cloves of garlic

1 tsp Turmeric powder

Salt

Kombu or kelp pieces (1-2)

Soak beans for at least 4-6 hours and discard the soaking water. Combine ingredients and bring to a boil, then let simmer for one hour. This soup can be served to your pet as dressing topping off usual diet or by itself.

APPENDIX B

10 FOODS TO NEVER FEED YOUR PET

• • • •

Animal fat/ skins

They are too high in saturated fats, especially if they are fried and seasoned. This is a big cause of pancreatitis in dogs and cats. About 1-2 days post ingestion they start severe vomiting or diarrhea which requires hospitalization.

Grapes

They are very toxic in any amount. The exact toxin is unknown but I've lost two patients (a skunk and a dog) after eating grapes and raisins despite having intravenous fluids and supportive care. This toxin causes the kidneys to shut down.

Chocolate

The chemical in it is theobromine which can be fatal to dogs and cats depending on the dose eaten and the purity of the chocolate. The darker the chocolate the more toxin it contains. This poisoning needs urgent veterinary care.

Macadamia nuts

The symptoms of macadamia nut poisoning are similar to any pancreatitis case; vomiting, anorexia and weakness. However, we see tremors and Central Nervous System signs as well. The toxin is not well known but keep your pups away from these nuts.

Corn cobs

These do not digest or break down in the gut so the dogs that bit big chunks of corn cobs end up having emergency surgery to remove it from the intestines.

Milk

Dogs and cats are lactose intolerant. Although cow milk itself is not really toxic, it is not in the best interest to give it to them. In addition, most dairy products like ice cream and yogurt are full of unhealthy sugars and fat and those could cause your pets to get pancreatitis.

Xylitol

This an artificial sweetener found in most diabetic friendly candy and sweets. It is also in some peanut butter products. This ingredient causes acute liver failure in pets and is extremely toxic in any amount.

Alcohol

Ethanol can cause signs of intoxication including incoordination and collapse. The severity of the symptoms corresponds to the amount ingested.

Avocados

Avocados are extremely fatty and could cause pancreatitis in sensitive pets, however the flesh is not poisonous to dogs and cats per se. The bark and pit of the avocado tree contains persin, a toxin for birds, horses, and wildlife.

Bread dough

Dough ingestion can be extremely deadly! It expands in the belly and can cause fatal blockages in their intestines. The yeast can ferment, releasing CO_2 gases and causing stomach bloat which is a real grave emergency.

APPENDIX C

TOP HERBAL FORMULAS

• • • •

THESE ARE FROM JING TANG HERBALS, INC. There are many other similar herbal formulas widely used by other TCVM practitioners. I just happen to have lots of success using these.

According to their website www.tcvmherbal.com "Jing Tang brand herbal products are distributed exclusively through licensed doctors for the best and safest care of the consumers. Over 200 Jing Tang brand formulas have been developed by Dr. Huisheng Xie, based on a history of 3000 years of traditional Chinese herbal recipe and his over 30 years of clinical experience."

Stasis Breaker (for cancer)

Is used to break down the masses through its action of removing the stagnation. The classical antecedent is the Chinese formula Nei Xiao Wan found in the text Wei Sheng Bio Jan (Precious Mirror of Health) written in 1279-1368 by Luo Tian Yi in Yuan dynasty. The ingredients and their actions are as follows;

Bai Hua She She Cao	Oldenandia	Inhibits cell mutation and tumor growth
Ban Zhi Lian	Scutellaria	Clear Heat-toxin, inhibits cell mutation and tumor growth
E Zhu Zedoaria	Purges the interior, break	Blood stasis and clear mass
Mu Li Ostrea	Softens hardness and clear mass	
San Leng Sparganium	Purges the interior, break stasis and clear mass	
Zhe Bei Mu Fritillaria	Softens hardness and clear nodules	

Liver Happy (for liver problems)

This herbal formula is a product from Jing Tang Herbals and its main indication is to relieve Liver *Qi* Stagnation. This is a version of the Classical Antecedent *Chai Hu Shu Gan* from Tai Ping Hui Min He Ji Ju Fang (Imperial Grace Formulary of the Tai Ping Era) written by Chen Shi-Wen et al in 1080. 4 The ingredients and their actions are as follows;

Bai Shao Yao	Paeonia = Soothe Liver
Bo He	Mentha = Move Qi
Chai Hu	Bupleurum = Soothe Liver
Chen Pi	Angelica = Move Blood
Dang Gui	Citrus = Dry up Dampness and Move Qi
Gan Cao	Glycyrrhiza = Harmonizer
Mu Dan Pi	Moutan = Cool Liver
Qing Pi	Citrus = Move Qi
Xiang Fu	Cyperus = Soothe Liver and resolve stagnation

Zhi Zi	Gardenia = Clear Heat
Wei Qi booster	(for cancer and immune disorders as well as energy booster)

Wei Qi booster main actions is to Tonifies *Qi* and Blood and increase the *Wei Qi* . It has antiviral, anticancer benefits thanks to the action of supporting normal cell division. The classical antecedent is *Si Jun Zi Tang* from Tai Ping Hui Min He Ji Ju Fang (Imperial Grace Formulary of the Tai Ping Era) written by Chen Shi Wen et al in 1080. These are the ingredients and their actions;

Bai Hua She She Cao	*Oldelandia*	Clears heat, inhibit cell mutation
Chen Pi	*Citrus*	Moves Qi, clears stagnation
Dan Gui	*Angelica*	Tonify, move blood, resolve stagnation
Dang Shen	*Codonopsis*	Tonify Qi
Huang Qi	*Astragalus*	Tonify Qi
Wu Yao	*Lindera*	Move Qi
Xuan Shen	*Scrophularia*	Resolve stagnation, nourish Yin
Ban Bian Lian	*Lobelia*	Clear heat

Double P (for paralysis)

Classical antecedent is Da Huo Luo Dan and the main indications is for Breaking down stasis in the spine. It also moves Qi thus resolving Stagnation. This can be a toxic formula and is used short term usually until enough progress in motor movement is gained.These are the ingredients and their actions;

Ba Ji Tian	Morinda	Tonify Kidney, strengthen bones
Bu Gu Zhi	Psoralea	Tonify Kidney, warms Spleen
Chi Sao	Paeonia	Resolves Stagnation
Chuang Xiong	Ligusticum	Move Qi and Blood, relieves pain
Dang Gui	Angelica	Nourishes Blood, relieves pain
Di Long	Pheretima	Detoxifies
Du Zhong	Eucommia	Strengthens back, Tonifies Kidney Yang
Fu Zi	Aconite	Warms Yang and Channels
Gan Cao	Glycyrrhiza	Harmonizes
Gu Sui Bu	Drynaria Tonifies	Kidney, Nourishes Liver, mends bones
Hong Hua	Carthamus	Resolves stagnation and stasis
Huang Qi	Astragalus	Tonifies Qi
Mo Yao	Myrrh	Resolves stagnation, relieves pain
Quan Xie	Buthus	Resolves stagnation
Ru Xiang	Olibanum	Moves Qi and blood, relieves pain
Tian San Qi	Notoginseng	Moves Blood, stops bleeding
Wu Gong	Scolopendra	Detoxifies
Wu Yao	Lindera	Move Qi, relieves pain
Xu Duan	Dipsacus	Strengthens bones and ligaments
Xue Jie	Draconis	Resolves Stagnation

Shen Calmer (insomnia, heart disease and behavioral disorders)

Nourishes the Heart Yin and Blood, calms Shen, and soothes the Liver Qi. Great formula for Anxiety & Insomnia Restlessness Nervousness Shen (spirit).

Ingredients and their actions;

Ostrea	Mu Li	Calms Shen subdues Liver Yang
Paeonia	Bai Shao Yao	Smoothes Liver Qi and Nourish Blood
Biota	Bai Zi Ren	Calms Shen nourish Heart
Angelica	Dang Gui	Nourishes Heart Blood
Ophiopogon	Mai Men Dong	Nourishes Heart Yin
Zizyphus	Suan Zao Ren	Calms Shen, nourishes Heart
Asparagus	Tian Men Dong	Nourishes Heart Yin
Cyperus	Xiang Fu Zi	Smoothes Liver Qi
Polygala	Yuan Zhi	Calms Shen, nourishes Heart
Bupleurum	Chai Hu	Regulates Liver Qi and relieves stress
Salvia	Dan Shen	Invigorates Blood, dispels Stasis
Poria	Fu Shen	Calms Shen
Scrophularia	Xuan Shen	Cools Blood Heat
Polygonum	Ye Jiao Teng	Calms Shen nourishes Heart
Citrus	Qing Pi	Smoothes Liver Qi
Schisandra	Wu Wei Zi	Consolidates body fluids

Body Sore (for pain)

This formula invigorates *Qi* and blood, resolves stagnation and relieves stagnation

Angelica	Dang Gui	Activates Blood, resolves & relieves stagnation
Corydalis	Yan Hu Suo	Move Qi/Blood, resolves & relieves stagnation
Paeonia	Chi Shao Yao	Relieves stagnation and cools Blood
Ligusticum	Chuan Xiong	Relieves stagnation and activate Blood
Angelica	Du Huo	Relieves Pain and eliminates Wind-Damp
Myrrh	Mo Yao	Moves Blood, relieves stagnation
Notopterygium	Qiang Huo	Relieves stagnation and activates blood
Olibanum	Ru Xiang	Moves Blood, relieves stagnation
Psoralea	Bu Gu Zhi	Strengthens bone and tonifies Yang
Cyathula	Chuan Niu Xi	Relieves stagnation and eliminates Wind-Damp
Eucommia	Du Zhong	Strengthens back and tonify Yang
Carthamus	Hong Hua	Breaks down Blood stasis, relieve stagnation
Millettia	Ji Xue Teng	Nourishes Blood
Persica	Tao Ren	Breaks down Blood stasis, relieves stagnation
Cuscuta	Tu Si Zi	Nourish Kidney and Liver
Epimedium	Yin Yang Huo	Tonifies Kidney Yang and Yin

Di tan tang (for seizures)

This formula transforms phlegm, clears internal Wind and stops seizures.

Citrus	Chen Pi	Move Qi, transforms phlegm
Arisema	Dan Nan Xing	Transforms phlegm
Acorus	Shi Chang Pu	open the orifice, eliminate Damp
Bambusa	Zhu Ru	Transform phlegm
Uncaria	Gou Teng	Extinguish Internal Wind, clear Liver Heat
Sargassum	Hai Zao	Transform Phlegm, clear Heat, soften the hardness
Laminaria	Kun Bu	Transform phlegm, soften the hardness, drain water
Haliotis	Shi Juen Ming	Clear Liver Heat
Poria	Fu Ling	Drain Damp
Aurantium	Zhi Shi	Move Qi
Ginseng	Ren Shen	Tonify Qi
Licorice	Gan Cao	Harmonize
Zingiberis	Gan Jiang	Harmonize

Tendon ligament (for knee injuries)

This formula nourishes Liver Yin and Blood, strengthen tendons and ligaments

Lycium	Gou Qi Zi	Nourish Liver Yin and Blood
Ligusticum	Chuan Xiong	Move Blood, resolve stagnation
Paeonia	Bai Shao Yao	Nourish Blood and Yin, soothe Liver Yang
Cornus	Shan Zhu Yu	Nourish Liver Yin
Acanthopanax	Wu Jia Pi	Strengthen ligaments and tendons

Achyranthes	Niu Xi	Strengthens the Kidney and benefits the knees
Rehmannia	Shu Di Huang	Nourish Blood and Yin
Psoler	Bu Gu Zhi	Nourish Kidney Yang and Yin
Epimedium	Yin Yang Huo	Nourish Kidney Yang and Yin
Angelica	Dang gui	Nourish Blood
Morus	Sang Zhi	Smoothen limbs
Cinnamon	Gui Zhi	Activate the Channels and limbs

Heart Qi tonic (for heart disease)

This formula tonifies the Heart Qi and invigorates Blood

Codonopsis	Dang Shen	Tonify Qi
Astragalus	Huang Qi	Tonify Qi
Licorice	Gan Cao	Tonify Qi
Poria	Fu Ling	Drains Damp
Lingusticum	Chuan Xiong	Moves Blood
Angelica	Dang Gui	Nourish Blood
Biota	Bai Zi Ren	Tonify Heart
Polygala	Yuan Zhi	Tonify Heart
Schisandra	Wu Wei Zi	Astringent
Cinnamon	Rou Gui	Warm Yang

APPENDIX D

HOW TO LOCATE A HOLISTIC VETERINARIAN?

• • • •

THE FOLLOWING WEBSITES CONTAIN lots of helpful information and also practitioner directories.

Chi Institute www.tcvm.com

International Veterinary Acupuncture Society www.ivas.org

American Academy of Veterinary Acupuncture www.aava.org

American Holistic Veterinary Medical Association www.ahvma.org

Academy of Veterinary Homeopathy http://theavh.org/

REFERENCES

• • • •

1. Xie,H., Ferguson,B., Xiaolin, D, Application of Tui-Na in Veterinary Medicine 2nd edition. Reddick, Fl Chi Institute of Chinese Veterinary Medicine. 2007 16,20,21,39

2. Xie,H., Preast, V. Traditional Chinese Veterinary Medicine Fundamental Principles 1st edition. Reddick, Fl Chi Institute of Chinese Veterinary Medicine. 2007 Appendix D

3. Chi Institute of Chinese Medicine, Small Animal Acupuncture Training Program. Wet Lab Handout, Spring Class 2010

4. Chi Institute of Chinese Medicine, Small Animal TCVM Diagnostics, Classical Points and Advanced Acupuncture Techniques. Wet Lab Handout, Spring Class 2012.

5. Xie, H., Chinese Veterinary Herbal Handbook. Ed. Vanessa Preast. 2nd ed. Reddick: Chi Institute of Chinese Medicine, 2008.

6. Chi Institute of Chinese Medicine, Small Animal TCVM Diagnostics, Veterinary Food Therapy Training program Handbook. Class 2010

9 781628 653922